A Shadow as Old as Time: A History of Cancer Through the Ages

Catherine

TABLE OF CONTENTS

Chapter 1: Introduction

1.1 Cancer Metastasis: history and epidemiology, biology, and clinical implications

History and Epidemiology

Unlike a majority of the diseases that humanity has encountered, succumbed to or overcame, cancer is a disease older than the human race and has always been prevalent in our history of medicine. The oldest known record of cancer is breast cancer (BC), described in the Edwin Smith Papyrus in 3000 BC as masses in the breast that are incurable.[1] The subsequent Ebers Papyrus, written in 1500 BC, further describes other tumors of the skin, uterus, and gastrointestinal tract.[1] The Greek physician Hippocrates (460-375 BC) is credited with coining the term "cancer", after associating the moving invasive protrusions of tumor masses to the claws of a crab.[1] Throughout antiquity, various cultures attempted to treat these masses with cauterization, crude surgery, bloodletting, salts, herbal remedies, and heavy metal poisons, practices that were often fatal and remained unchanged for over 3000 years until the advent of modern medicine.[1]

Although modern medicine has improved the survival rate of many cancer types, cancer remains the second leading cause of death in the USA.[2] It is estimated that 1,898,160 new cancer cases will be diagnosed in 2021 in the USA, with 608,570 patients succumbing to the disease.[2] The overall mortality rate of cancer patients is dependent on type of cancer, incidence, stage of diagnosis, and efficacy of available treatments.[2,3] For example, USA cancer mortality rates peaked in 1991 (215 cancer deaths per 100,000 cases) due to the smoking epidemic, which resulted in high incidences of lung cancer (until recently, the most common cancer), but a reduction in smoking habits have seen an improvement in both lung cancer mortality and overall cancer mortality.[2,3] Furthermore, numerous treatment breakthroughs have significantly reduced mortality in specific cancers, such as melanoma.[3] However, the progress for treating other cancers, such as BC, have slowed since the reduction in mortality due to implementation of early-screening procedures.[2,3] Nonetheless, regardless of cancer type and treatment, it is undeniable that metastatic disease remains the primary cause of cancer-related deaths.[4] In the clinic, cancer diagnosis and progression is typically classified into five stages, 0, I, II, III, and IV (Table 1-1).[5] Stage 0 is referred to as carcinoma in situ disease and generally describes non-malignant pre-cancerous lesions. Stage I represents localized cancer, in which the malignant tumor is small and localized in a single area without nodal or vascular spread. Stage II and III represent early and late locally/regional advanced cancer, in which tumor is large in size and has extensively invaded into regional tissues and lymph nodes.[5] Solid tumors of stages I-III are generally operable, with the chances of complete resection decreasing with increasing stage.[5] Stage IV metastatic disease, in which clinically detectable metastases have formed in distant organs, however, generally represents an incurable, manageable, and terminal disease.[2,5] It is well understood that about 90% of all cancer-related mortality is attributed to development of stage IV metastatic disease.[4] Indeed, the lethality of metastatic disease is reflected in the five-year survival rates for both high mortality cancers, such as pancreatic ductal adenocarcinoma (PDAC) (Stages I-III = 39-13%; Stage IV = 3%) and lung cancer (Stages I-III = 59-32%; Stage IV = 6%) and lower mortality cancers, such as BC (Stages I-III = 99-86%; Stage IV = 28%) and colon cancer (Stages I-III = 91-72%; Stage IV = 14%) (Table 1-1).[2]

Cancer Type	All Stages	Local	Regional	Distant
Breast	90	99	86	28
Colon	63	91	72	14
Rectum	67	89	72	14
Esophagus	20	47	25	5
Kidney	75	93	70	13
Larynx	61	78	45	34
Liver	20	34	12	3
Lung and bronchus	21	59	32	6
Melanoma	93	99	66	27
Oral cavity and pharynx	66	85	67	40
Ovary	49	93	75	30
Pancreas	10	39	13	3
Prostate	98	>99	96	73
Stomach	32	70	32	6
Testis	95	99	96	73
Thyroid	98	>99	98	55
Urinary bladder	77	69	37	6
Uterine cervix	66	92	58	17
Uterine corpus	81	95	69	17

Table 1-1: Five-year relative survival rates (%) by cancer stage at diagnosis, US, 2010-2016
Table showing the five-year relative survival rates of various cancer types from patient data from
SEER 18 from 2010-2018. Survival rates are shown as a % of patients surviving for five years
post-diagnosis and are stratified by all stages and stages at diagnosis: local (stage I), regional
(stages II-III), and distant disease (stage IV). Rates are based on cases diagnosed from SEER 18
locations from 2010-2016 and followed through 2017. Information source: Table 8, (American
Cancer Society, 2021)

Biology

Similar to the progression of cancer through its clinically defined stages, cancer metastasis represents a multistage progression of biological processes, which are collectively termed the metastatic cascade and first proposed by Irwin Bross in 1975.[4,6] The metastatic cascade describes the process of how malignant tumor cells 1) invade through the basement membrane of local tissue, 2) disseminate from the primary tumor, 3) intravasate, travel, and survive through circulation, 4) extravasate into the tissue of a distant organ, and finally 5) their escape from dormancy as either single tumor cells or micrometastases to proliferate and form clinically detectable and relevant malignant macroscopic metastatic (macrometastases) colonies (Figure 1-1).[4] The elucidation of the complex series of steps and mechanisms of the metastatic cascade is the result of many landmark experiments and observations by dedicated physicians and researchers.

The term, "metastasis", was first defined by the French physician, Joseph-Claude-Anthelme Récamier in 1829.[7] Récamier described the "transfer of cancer from one organ to another not directly connected to it" and hypothesized that invasion of tumor cells into circulation may be the route of disease spread.[7] In 1858, Rudolf Virchow, a Polish pathologist, proposed that metastases are formed from malignant cells that disseminate from the primary tumor through mechanical factors.[8] However, this was insufficient to determine the mechanism for how the disseminated cells seed into distant organs or explain how specific metastatic sites can vary from different types of cancers.

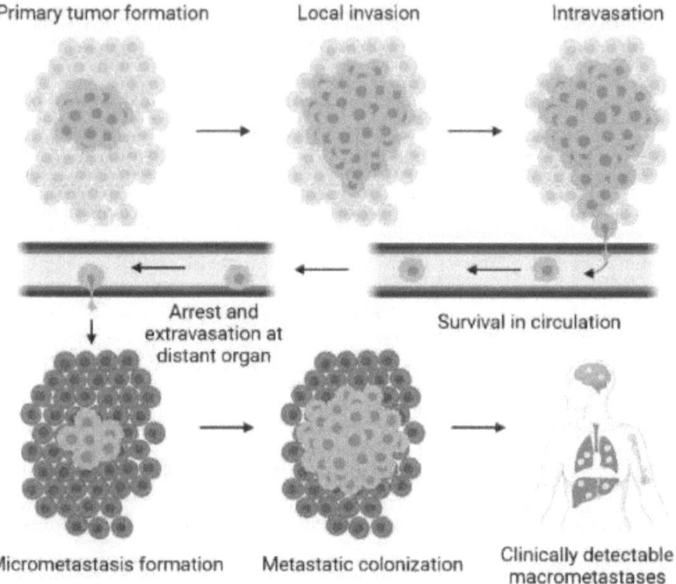

Figure 1-1: The metastatic cascade

The formation of clinically relevant metastases in distant organs represent the endpoint of a multitude of biological processes collectively described as the metastatic cascade. The metastatic cascade starts with tumor cells from the primary tumor invading into local tissue, intravasating into circulation, translocating and surviving through circulation, and arresting and extravasating into the parenchyma of distant organs. These tumor cells initially form small micrometastases that may remain indolent until they adapt organ-specific programs or modulate the host organ microenvironment to provide necessary survival and growth signals. Acquisition of these programs or signals then allow micrometastases to proliferate and form clinically detectable macroscopic metastases.

Upon the observation of BC patient autopsy records – which revealed that sites of metastasis were not random - Stephen Paget proposed the "seed and soil" hypothesis in 1889.[9] The hypothesis states that metastatic colonization is organ specific and not random; and that metastatic "seeds" can only grow in congenial "soil", in which the seed is the cancer cell and the soil is the microenvironment of the secondary organ.[9] The hypothesis stresses that cancer cell-host organ microenvironment interaction is critical for the formation of metastases and metastases only form if both seed and soil are compatible.[10] Indeed, many cancers exhibit organ-specific metastatic colonization. For example, colorectal cancer (CRC) and PDAC frequently metastasize to the liver, and lungs to a lesser extent, but rarely to bone, skin, or brain.[11] However, BC metastasizes to the bone, lungs, liver, and brain; and prostate cancer metastasizes to the bone, but rarely to the lung and liver.[11]

Paget's theory was challenged in 1929 by James Ewing, who argued that metastatic dissemination occurs only by mechanical factors dependent on the anatomic structure of vasculature.[10,11] An example of this is that in CRC and PDAC, the liver is the most common metastatic site because blood flow from the pancreas and gastrointestinal tract flows directly to the liver, resulting in the massive influx and deposition of tumor cells into the liver and leading to the formation of liver metastases.[2] Indeed, extensive experimental pathological analysis by Dale Rex Coman revealed that metastases do derive from tumor cell arrest in capillary beds: a vascular-mechanical phenomena.[10] However, Balduin Lucke demonstrated through experimental intravenous injections of metastatic V_2 rabbit carcinoma into either the portal vein/hepatic artery or systemic vein that metastatic growth was always higher in the liver compared to lung, and was independent of injection route.[12] This suggested that while tumor cell arrest is a vascular event, metastatic growth rates are organ specific.[12] Indeed, review of clinical data regarding metastatic sites of various cancers by Sugarbaker in 1979 revealed that while common regional metastases can be derived by anatomical/mechanical factors, metastases to distant organs were site specific in many cancer types.[10,13]

This was soon followed by Isiah Fidler's landmark experiment, in which he grafted lung, ovary, and kidney tissues into syngeneic mice and injected highly metastatic B16-F10 melanoma cells intravenously into engrafted mice.[10,14] While all three organs grafted successfully, Fidler observed that the B16 cells metastasized preferentially to the lungs and ovaries but not the kidneys, despite the fact that the anatomical vascularization between all engrafted organs were identical.[14] Fidler also analyzed the initial arrest of tumor cells at ten minutes, one hour, and one day post-injection and revealed that there was no significant difference in the number of tumor cells that arrested between engrafted lungs and kidneys in any of these early timepoints.[14] This study confirmed that while anatomical-mechanical factors do play a role in the initial arrest of tumor cells into distant organs, tumor cells indeed preferentially grow and metastasize in specific organs, thus validating Paget's theory.[14] A following study by Fidler demonstrated that isolating cancer cells that have metastasized *in vivo* and reimplanting them into mice increased the metastatic ability of the cells upon each successive cycle of isolation and re-engraftment.[15] Moreover, the experiment showed that selected "highly metastatic" cancer cells (following multiple selection cycles) display higher rates of survival in distant organs when compared to the "lowly metastatic" parental line, further demonstrating that metastasis is a selective process and tumor cell-host organ interaction is critical for metastasis.[15,16]

Fidler also revealed through intravenous injection of ^{125}I-5-iodo-2'-deoxyuridine-labeled B16 melanoma cells into syngeneic mice that only about 1% of all injected tumor cells survived after 24 hours, with approximately 400 individual cells capable of developing into an average of

78 metastatic colonies.[17] This demonstrated that while 1) metastasis is a highly inefficient process, with the vast majority tumor cells dying in circulation, and 2) few individual tumor cells from a tumor have the ability to metastasize; only a few tumor cells are necessary to form metastatic colonies.[17] Moreover, subsequent studies found that tumor cells that metastasize to specific organs display unique gene expression alterations that favor metastasis to the distant organ, which is consistent with previous findings that highly metastasis tumor cells can be selected for by multiple cycles of engraftment, isolation of cells from metastases, and rengraftment.[18] These studies reveal that successful metastasis is dependent on a tumor's clonal population of tumor-initiating cells, their seeding potential, and their ability to adopt organ-specific colonization programs.

However, questions remain regarding the molecular mechanisms of how tumor cells can acquire motility and invasive properties. In 2002, upon observation of how an epithelial-mesenchymal transition (EMT) reprograming of cells can confer upon epithelial cells the mobility of mesenchymal cells during development or wound healing; Thiery and Weinberg hypothesized that this EMT program could similarly allow cancer cells to acquire invasive properties.[4,19,20] Subsequent studies have shown that this EMT program is a partial alteration, in which epithelial tumor cells lose some of their epithelial traits, such as E-cadherin-mediated cell to cell adhesion, and acquire some mesenchymal traits, resulting in increased motility, invasiveness, and the ability to degrade extracellular matrix (ECM) components.[4] Indeed, circulating tumor cells (CTCs) from BC patients were found to express both epithelial and mesenchymal markers, while primary tumor cells contained mostly epithelial markers, suggesting that partial EMT plays a role in the dissemination of tumor cells.[21] Further studies have revealed that EMT is orchestrated by the master-regulator transcription factors, Snail, Slug, Twist, and Zeb1, and the expression of these can be induced by a variety of cytokines, growth factors, and signaling pathways, such as Wnt.[4]

Although formal proof that EMT is necessary or absolutely required to establish metastases is lacking, there is compelling evidence that EMT programs do promote metastatic potential in tumor cells when activated.

Successful metastatic colonization is also dependent on the presence or development of a supportive microenvironment niche in the host organ. Tumor cells that have disseminated into a distant organ naturally find themselves in a novel microenvironment with differing stromal cells, immune cells, growth factors, and ECM composition compared to their primary site. Keith Luzzi demonstrated using intraportal injection of B16 melanoma cells that while 80% of injected cells survived injection and extravasated into the liver, 36% of these remained as individual cells.[22] Additionally, 1 in 40 extravasated cells formed micrometastases, with only 1% of all micrometatases progressing to form macrometatases.[22] Interestingly, 95% of the individual surviving cells and several micrometastases were found to be in a state of non-proliferating dormancy and could persist as indolent cells for months and years, only to exit dormancy when favorable conditions are met.[22] This would explain the phenomena of residual cancer burden (RCB), also known as minimal residual disease (MRD), and relapse, in which a small number of cancer cells that have either seeded to distant organs or remain in the primary location after successful surgical or anti-neoplastic treatment have removed the primary tumor.[4] These dormant tumor cell(s) can eventually adapt organ-specific programs or modulate the host microenvironment, including mechanisms such as angiogenesis or immunomodulation, to exit dormancy and form clinically relevant macrometastases, a process that may take years.[22]

Clinical Implications

As stated previously, stage IV metastatic disease represents the terminal stage of cancer and the cause of 90% of all cancer-associated mortality.[4] The deadly nature of metastases stems from their 1) local effects, such as organ failure due to gross metastatic burden, 2) distribution throughout multiple organs, 3) decreased sensitivity and increased resistance to radiation therapy (RT) and chemotherapy compared to the primary tumor, 4) dormancy programs allowing for tumor cells to escape detection and treatment by anti-neoplastic agents, and 5) systemic effects that compromise the host's natural homeostasis (Figure 1-2). These systemic effects can result in dysregulated immune response and metabolism both promote tumor growth, survival, and invasion and render the host more susceptible to other co-morbidities and decreased tolerance to anti-neoplastic agents.

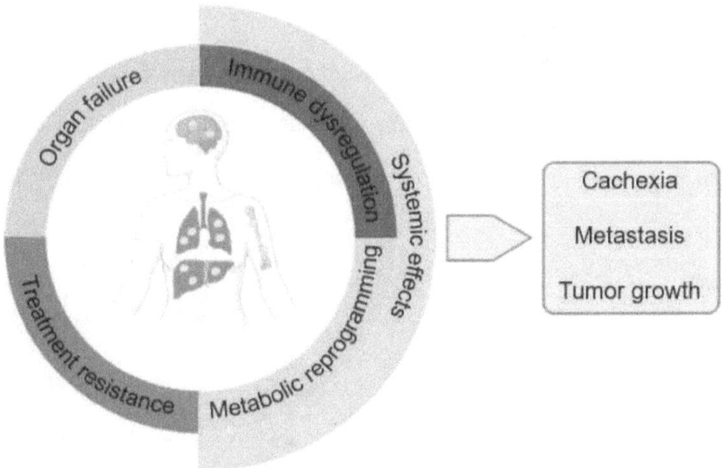

Figure 1-2: The effects of cancer metastasis

Overview of the effects of cancer metastasis that contribute to cancer-associated mortality.

Local Effects

The local effects of metastases-associated deaths are relatively straightforward and have been understood since antiquity. The growth of a malignant mass represents a physical barrier that interferes and damages the body's anatomy. The unrestrained growth of a tumor mass within an organ will compromise the function of said organ and result in organ failure. Furthermore, the mass can restrict blood vessels and circulation, neuron circuitry, respiratory function, and digestive tract function. In this manner, metastases can cause death by physically interference of the host's internal anatomical tissues and their functions. Therefore, the number of different and specific organ(s) bearing metastases can significantly impact patient survival and prognosis.[23] For example, BC patients bearing brain and multi-site metastases have significantly lower survival compared to those with lung-only and liver-only metastases, with bone-only metastatic patients having the best prognosis.[23] The local effects of metastasis are generally more lethal than that the primary tumor, because the primary tumor is generally localized to a singular location and in many early-stage cancers, can be surgically removed. However, metastatic disease is widespread, more difficult to detect, and often presents in vital and sensitive organs difficult to access through surgical means.

Treatment resistance

Since Emil Grubbé first pioneered RT treatment of cancer patients in 1933, it is estimated that over 50% of cancer patients receive RT during the course of their disease.[24-26] However, while RT remains effective in treating primary tumors, it known that RT can also promote metastasis.[24] RT can cause tumor, immune, and stromal cells to secrete metastasis-promoting cytokines, growth factors, and ECM-remodeling proteins.[24] Furthermore, distant tissues exposed to radiation through RT have been found to exhibit an increased propensity for metastatic colonization, which is mediated by radiation-induced hypoxia, damage to tissue vasculature, and pro-tumor inflammation.[24] Furthermore, RT treatment has also been shown to increase the number of CTCs, suggesting a role of RT in tumor cell dissemination from the primary tumor.[24] Finally, prolonged RT acts as a selecting agent for radioresistant clones that display an increased metastatic potential, which can result in relapse that is resistant to RT.[24]

Chemotherapy remains a mainstay of systemic anti-neoplastic treatment. Although their specific mechanisms differ, chemotherapeutic agents generally target various phases and mechanisms in the cell cycle to kill fast-dividing cells. While this is effective in killing rapidly proliferating tumor cells, dormant disseminated tumor cells in MRD can effectively bypass chemotherapeutic intervention by halting its cell cycle.[27] Another major issue in chemotherapy is intrinsic or acquired drug resistance; and it is estimated that 90% of chemotherapy failure occurs during the invasion and metastasis stages of cancer.[28] Furthermore, even successful treatment of the primary tumor by either RT or chemotherapy can result in later metastatic outgrowth that is resistant to the initial treatment. For example, while chemotherapy is able to manage early stage BC, treatment loses efficacy in the 30% of patients that progress to metastatic disease.[29] Only 30-70% of these patients respond to first line anthracycline or taxane chemotherapy and their median progression-free survival (mPFS) is limited to 6-10 months before onset of chemoresistance.[29] Patients resistant to first line treatment are then treated with capecitabine, but the response rates and mPFS drops significantly to 15-28% and < 6 months, respectively.[29,30] Similar trends are observed in other cancers, such as locally advanced rectal cancer, in which combined chemoradiation therapy fails in the 25-40% of patients that develop distant metastases; and advanced ovarian cancer, in which 80% of patients that respond well to first line chemotherapy ultimately relapse, with only 15-35% of patients responding to second line therapy.[31,32] This suggests that tumor acquisition of drug resistance is a selective and progressive process. Indeed, studies have shown that drug resistance can be caused by a variety of intrinsic, such as tumor heterogeneity and selection of resistant variants, and multi-drug resistance (MDR) mechanisms (e.g. drug efflux, drug metabolism, and inhibition of apoptosis), and extrinsic factors, such as modulation of the tumor microenvironment (TME) and inducing non-cancer cells to release pro-tumor survival factors.[28,33]

It is well known that tumors masses are heterogeneous, and this intra-tumor heterogeneity contains a multitude of tumor cell variants with alterations in their genetic (e.g. mutations, gene amplifications, aneuploidy, and translocations), epigenetic (e.g. chromosomal and histone modifications, hyper/hypomethylation, and hyper/hypoacetylation), transcriptomic, and proteomic backgrounds.[28] Moreover, tumor cells exhibit a high rate of genetic instability and aneuploidy, leading to high mutation and chromosomal rearrangement rates that can drive the development of novel drug-resistant variants.[28,34] Because chemotherapy acts as a selecting agent for tumor cells that have acquired various mechanisms of chemoresistance, over the course of treatment, these resistant variants gradually become the predominant population and this ultimately results in treatment failure.

In addition, because there is overlap between mechanisms conferring drug resistance and mechanisms involved in invasion and metastasis, such as EMT, drug resistant variants often have increased metastatic potential and thus their metastases are intrinsically resistant.[33,35] One such mechanism is through upregulation of Twist, a transcription factor that promotes EMT and metastasis, which can also upregulate the expression of P-glycoprotein (P-gp).[35,36] P-gp is an ATP-dependent membrane efflux transporter that contributes to MDR by binding to a multitude of chemotherapeutic agents (e.g. taxol, doxorubicin, etoposide, and paclitaxel) and utilizes ATP to release them into extracellular space.[28,37,38] Other mechanisms linking metastasis and MDR have

been observed in amplified drug metabolism and inhibition of apoptosis.[32,39,40] Studies have also

demonstrated that elevated glutathione S-transferase (GST) and glutathione (GSH), which confer

MDR through detoxification of drugs (e.g. cyclophosphamide, adriamycin, and cisplatin) and

ionizing molecules (e.g. reactive oxygen species), correlate directly with liver metastatic potential

in B16 melanoma.[35,39,41] Moreover, GST can indirectly inhibit drug-induced apoptosis pathways

via inhibition of mitogen-activated protein kinase (MAPK), c-Jun N-terminal kinase 1 (JNK1),

and apoptosis signal-regulating kinase 1 (ASK1).[39,40] Furthermore, elevated expression of

aldehyde dehydrogenase (ALDH), which detoxifies and confers resistance to a multitude of drugs

(e.g. cyclophosphamide, cisplatin, doxorubicin, taxanes, and temozolomide), has also been shown

to correlate with metastatic capability.[42] Elevated ALDH expression has been shown in both

clinical studies and multiple mouse cancer models, including BC, prostate cancer, ovarian cancer,

and hepatic cancer, to play a functional role in metastasis.[42] These studies, along with a multitude

of others, demonstrate that metastasis and intrinsic tumor chemoresistance pathways are linked.

However, metastasis and chemoresistance are also linked via extrinsic factors as well.

Similar to RT, chemotherapy is a systemic treatment that acts as a stress-inducer that promotes

tissue damage, hypoxia, and dysregulated stromal and immune responses that can favor

metastasis.[33,43] Studies of prostate cancer show that chemotherapy induces stromal cells to secrete

Wnt ligands, which then drives tumor cell EMT and metastasis.[42] Studies in lung cancer show that

chemotherapy induces cancer-associated fibroblasts (CAFs) to secrete growth factors, such as

IGF-1, HGF-1, and SDF-1, which promote tumor cell survival, proliferation, and EMT.[44] Our

laboratory has also demonstrated that chemotherapy drugs (e.g. doxorubicin and

cyclophosphamide) induce stromal cells to secrete TNF-α, which then induces BC cells to secrete

CXCL1. [45] CXCL1 then recruits neutrophils that secrete S100A8/9 cytokines that promote both primary tumor and metastatic BC cell survival and drug resistance through activation of ERK1/2 pathways.[45] Inhibition of this mechanism significantly reduces lung metastasis and increases the efficacy of chemotherapy.[45] Other studies have also shown that chemotherapy can "prime" certain tissue microenvironments to be more permissible to tumor cell intra and extravasation, which supports metastatic colonization.[33] These studies, along with others, demonstrate that chemotherapy treatment can promote metastasis by modulation of extrinsic factors, thus limiting the long-term efficacy of treatment.

In addition to RT and chemotherapy, targeted therapeutics are also utilized in the treatment of cancers, although their usage is highly dependent on cancer type and expression of drug target. While targeted therapeutics generally represent a more efficient option and are less harmful to the host compared to systemic chemotherapy, most treatments share similar challenges of acquired resistance and reduced efficacy in metastatic patients. An example is with kinase inhibitors, such as erlotinib and vemurafenib, which are used to treat EGFR-mutant lung cancer and BRAF-mutant melanoma patients, respectively. Initial treatment is usually successful with partial to full tumor regression, however the duration until acquisition of resistance, tumor progression, and metastasis is a low 6-12 months.[46] Subsequent experimental studies using mouse and xenograft models revealed that while the tumor and TME regressed upon treatment, the treatment stimulated stressed melanoma and lung cancer cells, which ultimately promoted the proliferation, invasion, and metastasis of resistant tumor cells.[46] Targeted endocrine therapy, such as tamoxifen, in estrogen receptor (ER)-positive BC is another example of acquisition of resistance in recurrence and metastasis.[47] Studies show that around 33% of treated patients acquire resistance, many of them through mutations in the ER coding gene, *ESR1*.[47] These ER-mutant tumor cells were found to be significantly higher in metastases than in primary tumors, suggesting that acquisition of ER resistance is linked to metastasis.[47] Taken altogether, these studies link metastasis to resistance to radio, chemo, and targeted therapeutic intervention, further underscoring the lethal nature of metastatic disease and the pressing need to discover novel targetable mechanisms for the treatment of metastatic patients.

1.2 Metastasis and Immunotherapy – background, state of the field, new frontiers – B cells

Background

Throughout the initiation and progression of both primary tumors and their metastases, tumor cells will interact with the host's immune system. The growth, survival, and metastasis of tumor cells is intricated linked to tumor-immune crosstalk and the balance between anti-tumor and pro-tumor inflammation and immune cell phenotypes.[48] It is well understood that cytotoxic CD8$^+$ T lymphocytes (CTLs) and natural killer cells (NK) cells mediate anti-tumor immunity and depletion of these populations result in increased formation of metastasis in various mouse models of cancer.[48-52] Conventionally, anti-tumor immune response requires tumor cells to express neoantigens/tumor-associated antigens (TAA), which are internalized by antigen-presenting cells (APCs), such as dendritic cells (DCs) or B cells, and displayed on their surface MHC-I or MHC-II proteins. These APCs then migrate to the TME or draining lymph nodes through locally-released inflammatory cytokines and chemokines where they present the TAAs to CTLs. This primes the CTLs to secrete pro-inflammatory cytokines, recognize TAA-expressing tumor cells, and kill the malignant cells through release of perforin and granzyme B.[48] There is extensive evidence that decreased tumor CTL infiltration is associated with poor prognosis in many cancer types, including

BC, ovarian, and CRC; and depletion of CTLs in mouse models of results in increased metastasis.[49,50,53-56] NK cells target tumor cells deficient in MHC-I and studies in multiple mouse models of cancer show that NK cell depletion can increase metastasis.[51,57,58] Myeloid cells, such as macrophages and neutrophils, can also mediate anti-tumor functions through phagocytosis and secretion of reactive oxygen species (ROS), although their phenotypes are often found to be altered to a tumor-promoting role.[48]

Tumor cells must evade these anti-tumor response mechanisms to successfully grow and metastasize. One method is through establishment of an immunosuppressive TME through the release of tumor-derived cytokines, such as TGF-β or IL-10, which can trigger the differentiation of anti-tumor immune cells into a pro-tumor immune phenotype, such T-regulatory cells (Tregs), tumor-associated macrophages (TAMs), and tumor-associated neutrophils (TANs).[59-62] These immunosuppressive immune cells secrete immunosuppressive cytokines and express T cell co-inhibitory molecules to blunt CTL-mediated anti-tumor response.[48] Tregs, TAMs, and TANs have all been demonstrated to promote metastasis in mouse models of BC through the suppression of anti-tumor immune responses.[45,63,64] Furthermore, the secretion of tumor- or TME-derived cytokines, such as G-CSF, into systemic circulation alters the hematopoiesis and generation of myeloid cells in the bone marrow, resulting in both local and systemic accumulation of immunosuppressive TANs and immature myeloid-derived suppressor cells (MDSCs).[48] This creates a systemic "myeloid-bias" skewing of immune homeostasis, which promotes the survival of tumor cells in circulation and promotes the formation of pre-metastatic niches in distant organs that promotes metastatic colonization. Immunosuppressive immune cells have also been shown to promote metastasis through secretion or expression of ECM remodeling proteins, such as matrix metalloproteinases, and angiogenesis-stimulating proteins, such as VEGF-A, which increase the invasion and intra/extravasation of tumor cells, respectively.[48] Moreover, ECM and vascular remodeling can result in a high-density, fibrotic TME and leaky vasculature, respective, which can impair the infiltrating of anti-tumor immune cell populations.[48,65,66] Another method for tumor immune escape is for tumor cells and tumor-induced immunosuppressive immune cells to regulate their expression of inhibitory immunoreceptors (also known as immune checkpoints), such as PD-L1, CTLA-4, LAG3, and TIM3.[67,68] The binding of these immune checkpoint molecules to their cognate ligands, such as tumor PD-L1 to CTL PD-1, or T cell CTLA-4 to APC-CD80, will inactivate the CTL and revert it into an anergic state incapable of mediating anti-tumor response.[48,67,68]

State of the Field

Since the discovery of immune checkpoints in cancer, there has been an extensive effort in the research and development of antibody-based immune checkpoint inhibitors (ICIs) to increase T cell-mediated anti-tumor response. This has led to the FDA approval of many ICI treatments, including those targeting CTLA-4 (ipilimumab), PD-1 (pembrolizumab and nivolumab), and PD-L1 (atezolizumab, avelumab, and durvalumab).[69] These ICI therapies have yielded positive indications in a wide range of cancers, including, but not limited to, metastatic melanoma, lymphomas, renal cancer, and lung cancer.[69] However, the response and efficacy of ICIs are not universal, as ICIs have minimal efficacy in metastatic PDAC, metastatic castration-resistant prostate cancer, and metastatic triple-negative breast cancer (mTNBC).[69,70] Indeed, similar to tumor acquisition of resistance to other treatment discussed previously, tumors undergoing ICI treatment can develop mechanisms to escape T cell-mediated targeting. These mechanisms can include alterations in antigen presentation pathways, reduced CTL proliferation and diversity, downregulation of TAAs, increased immunosuppression in the TME, resistance to CTL effector molecules, and alterations in vasculature and ECM remodeling to reduce CTL infiltration into the TME.[69]

Clinical studies in BC patients show that metastases exhibit reduced CTL infiltrate, reduced pro-inflammatory cytokines and increased immunosuppressive cytokines, and decreased antigen presentation when compared to matched primary tumors.[71] This suggests that metastases are more immunologically inert and are more resistant to ICI.[71] This difference could explain the reduced mPFS of Atezolizumab in mTNBC (mPFS=6.6 months) when compared to locally advanced TNBC (mPFS=9.6 months).[70] The treatment efficacy of ICIs is not only dependent on whether the patient has developed metastases or not, but also on the number and sites of metastasis as well: atezolizumab: brain (mPFS=4.9 months), bone (mPFS=5.7 months), liver (mPFS=5.3 months), lung (mPFS=5.7 months); pembrolizumab: 0-3 sites (mPFS=8.0 months), >3 sites (mPFS=5.9 months).[70] Furthermore, atezolizumab efficacy is also dependent on its administration as a first or second-line treatment, as the overall response rate (ORR) in mTNBC falls from 24% as first-line treatment to 6% as second-line treatment.[72] This suggests that resistance mechanisms acquired during first-line treatment using other drugs can also play a role in ICI resistance, further decreasing the benefit of ICIs in an advanced metastatic disease context. This demonstrates a need for the discovery of other immunotherapies for the management of metastatic disease.

Another T cell-based immunotherapy is chimeric antigen receptor T cell (CAR-T) therapy, in which autologous T cells are taken from a patient, genetically engineered to express a synthetic T cell receptor (TCR) targeting a specific TAA, expanded *in vitro*, and injected back into the patient.[73] However, while CAR-T therapy is FDA-approved and efficacious in managing hematological malignancies, such as leukemia and lymphomas, they illicit poorer responses in solid tumors.[74] This lack of efficacy can be due to the difficultly in identifying TAAs, impaired CTL trafficking, a heavily immunosuppressive TME, and the heterogenous nature of solid tumors and selection of variants not expressing the specifically targeted TAA.[74]

Other immunotherapies that target myeloid cells are also actively being explored, albeit to limited efficacy in clinical trials when compared to preclinical mouse models. For example, blockade of CSF1/CSFR1 or CCL2/CCR2, which mediate TAM differentiation and recruitment, respectively, in combination with ICI failed to show benefit over chemotherapy in clinical trials.[75,76] Targeting of other macrophage targets, such as the SIRPα/CD47 phagocytosis-inhibition axis, have shown promising activity and response (36% complete response) in B cell malignancies in conjunction with anti-CD20 (rituximab).[77] However, efficacy in solid tumors remains low.[78,79] Phase I studies of anti-CCL2 (carlumab) in multiple solid tumors, including BC, showed only short duration transient suppression of free CCL2 with only 4/44 patients achieving response. Furthermore, a Phase IIb clinical trial of carlumab in metastatic castration-resistant prostate cancer showed ineffective blockade of CCL2/CCR2 signaling and no single-agent anti-tumor activity. Subsequent studies reveal that a pertinent issue with targeting TAMs in solid tumors is that although they do contribute to maintaining an immunosuppressive TME, there are a plethora of other immune cells, such as Tregs and TANs, that are functionally redundant. Furthermore, targeting TAM differentiation or trafficking does not directly mediate anti-tumor killing and upregulation of redundant pathways or cessation of treatment will restore TME TAM populations and result in continuation of tumor progression. Studies using patient samples and TNBC mouse models also revealed that cessation of anti-CCL2 treatment promotes TNBC lung metastasis, which is mediated by accelerated angiogenesis through upregulation of IL-6 and VEGF-A.[80] Zoledronic acid, which is used to strengthen bones in early BC patients, plays a role in reprogramming TAMs into anti-tumor M1 macrophages.[81] However, despite initial promise in early hormone-responsive BC patients observed in the phase III ABCSG-12 and ZO-FAST clinical trials, results from other phase III AZURE and SUCCESS A clinical trials revealed no significant reduction in disease-free survival (DFS), overall survival (OS), or bone metastases.[82,83]

Similarly, immunotherapies targeting immunosuppressive MDSCs are also being tested in clinical studies, with limited results. Entinostat is a class I histone deacetylase inhibitor with a role in reducing MDSC populations through epigenetic reprogramming.[84] However, entinostat failed to demonstrate increased mPFS in TNBC and ovarian cancer patients in the ENCORE 602 and ENCORE 603 clinical trials, respectively.[84] A CXCR1/CXC2R2 inhibitor, SX-682, that blocks recruitment of CXCR2$^+$ MDSCs has shown efficacy in combination with ICI in preclinical models, but is still currently undergoing phase I clinical trials.[84] Ibrutinib, a bruton's tyrosine kinase (BTK) inhibitor used in B cell malignancies that also targets BTK signaling-dependent macrophages and MDSCs, has also shown promising results in inhibiting tumor growth and metastasis in preclinical mouse models of BC and TNBC by converting MDSCs into DCs and enhancing CTL activity.[85-87] However, the phase III RESOLVE and phase Ib/II NCT02403271 clinical trials showed that ibrutinib in combination with chemotherapy or ICI yielded no improvement in mPFS or OS in metastatic PDAC patients, and poor ORR (3%) in advanced and metastatic HER2$^+$ and TNBC patients, respectively.[88]

Taken together, while immunotherapeutic intervention remains a novel and promising field in the management of primary tumors and metastatic disease, there are many limitations to its efficacy, especially in a metastatic context. Given the lethality of stage IV metastatic disease and its augmented resistance to current RT, chemotherapy, targeted therapies, and immunotherapy strategies, it is of vital important to elucidate novel metastasis-promoting mechanisms for potential targeting.

New Frontier – B cells

While the role of tumor-infiltrating myeloid cells and T lymphocytes have been extensively explored, the role and function of tumor-infiltrating B lymphocytes (TIBs) are less defined. However, there is growing interest in the functional roles of TIBs, as studies have demonstrated the presence of TIBs in about 70% of solid primary tumors, including PDAC, CRC, melanomas, and BC.[89,90] B cells are an integral part of the immune system. Although their canonical role is mediating humoral immunity through the production of antibodies, B cells also represent a heterogenous population that can mediate cellular immunity by secreting cytokines, performing effector functions, serving as professional APCs, acting as positive and negative regulators of myeloid and T cells, and maintenance of lymphoid tissues.[91]

Mature B cells are divided into three primary subsets: B1 cells, which are distinct from conventional B2 cells and located in the peritoneum and pleural cavities, B2 follicular (FO) B cells, located and comprising about 95% of the B cell population in secondary lymphoid organs (SLOs) and B2 marginal zone (MZ) B cells, located in the spleen's marginal zone.[92] B1 and MZ B cells are activated in a T cell independent manner, in which non-protein or crosslinked antigens are recognized by multiple B cell receptors (BCRs), and subsequently proliferate and differentiate into short lived immunoglobulin (Ig) producing plasma cells (PCs). FO B cells are activated in a T cell dependent manner, in which an antigen recognized by the BCR is internalized, fragmented, and presented on the FO B cell's MHC class II receptors to the TCRs of CD4$^+$ T helper cells. Upon successful recognition and in conjunction with the co-stimulatory FO B cell CD40 binding to CD4$^+$

T cell CD40L, the CD4[+] T cell then releases cytokines, IL-4 and IL-21, to activate and stimulate the FO B cell. The activated B cell then proliferates and differentiates into either short-lived PCs and effector B cells, or migrates to the germinal center (GC) of SLOs to become GC B cells. GC B cells undergo clonal expansion, somatic hypermutation, Ig class switching, and affinity selection to become either long-lived PCs with high affinity Ig secretion or memory cells.[92]

Several mechanisms of B cell recruitment to TME have been reported. Activated stromal cells in the TME can induce tissue-specific expression of CCL21 and CXCL13, which can recruit TIBs through their cognate B cell receptors, CCR7 and CXCR5, respectively.[89] Furthermore, tumor-associated blood vessels can also express CCL21; and tumor-associated TGF-β can also induce CD8[+] T cells to secrete CXCL13.[89] In solid tumors, TIBs have been found to be distributed as either singular cells at the invasive margin and the peritumoral stroma, or as aggregates within tertiary lymphoid structures (TLSs) or lymphocyte clusters (LCs).[90,93] TLSs share morphological and phenotypical similarities to SLOs and contain their own B cell follicles and functional GCs that can produce memory B cells and long-lived PCs.[94] Conventional SLO development requires hematopoietic lymphoid tissue inducer (LTi) cells that express membrane-bound lymphotoxin$\alpha_1\beta_2$ (LT) that binds to stromal tissue organizer cells to express adhesion molecules, such as ICAM1 and VCAM1, and maintain a lymphoid-chemokine feedback axis. This axis produces CCL19, CCL21, and CXC13, which recruit and segregate B and T cells and induce the differentiation of high endothelial venules.[94] While TLS formation is largely dependent on LT signaling, TLS can form without specific LTi cells as M1 macrophages and B and T cells can upregulate LT expression and drive TLS development upon CCL21 and CXCL13 signaling, respectively.[94] In particular, LT-expressing B cells, through CXCL13 signaling and interactions that induce stromal cell chemokine production, are critical to the formation and maintenance of B cell follicles in both SLOs and TLS.[94]

Interestingly, the presence of TLSs have been demonstrated to correlate with good prognosis in cancer patients and anti-tumor function in mouse models.[95-97] TLS-associated B cell (TLS-B) aggregates were found to be present in 37.69% of stage I-III BC patient primary tumors and correlated with increased distant disease-free survival (DDFS) (HR=0.251) and increased OS (HR=0.325) in hormone-negative patients.[98] High primary tumor TLS-B cell density is also correlated with improved metastasis-free survival and mOS in melanoma, gastric cancer, ovarian cancer, non-small cell lung cancer, hepatocellular carcinoma, Merkel cell carcinoma, bladder cancer, and CRC.[99-111] Furthermore, a recent clinical study revealed that elevated numbers of spatially dispersed LC-associated B cells (LC-B) in TNBC primary tumors correlate with good prognosis and increased recurrence/relapse-free survival (RFS) after initial treatment and mastectomy.[93]

Contrary to the positive correlation with TLS and prognosis, studies have shown that non-TLS TIBs have been associated with poor prognosis and tumor-promoting function. In PDAC patients, the prognostic value of TIBs is highly dependent on their spatial distribution as TLS-B or single TIBs.[97] A high TLS-B to TIB ratio was found to correlate with increased CTL cell infiltration and increased patient mOS (mOS=30.9 months) compared to patients with a low TLS-B to TIB ratio (mOS=14.1 months).[97] Furthermore, depletion of TIBs in allograft Pan02 and LSL-Kras^{G12D}-Pdx1-Cre genetically-modified mouse models (GEMM) of PDAC with an anti-CD20 antibody slightly reduced tumor size and increased CTL and NK cell infiltration, suggesting that singular TIBs have a pro-tumor function.[97] Other studies report that allograft implantation of EL4 thymoma, MC38 colon cancer, and B16 melanoma cell lines in syngeneic IgM$^{-/-}$ B cell-deficient mice (B-deficient) resulted in no tumor growth, spontaneous tumor regression after 10 days post inoculation, and significantly slowed tumor growth, respectively, compared to immunocompetent B cell-proficient (B-proficient) mice.[112] This increased resistance to tumor growth was attributed to elevated anti-tumor IFN-y and IL-12 cytokine concentrations and CTL response in B-deficient mice. Adoptive transfer of B cells from syngeneic mice into B-deficient mice lowered anti-tumor cytokine levels and CTL responses and restored tumor growth, indicating that B cells can inhibit anti-tumor responses in multiple histologically distinct murine tumor models.[112]

B cells have been implicated in tumorigenesis as well. TIBs have been reported to be the dominant lymphocyte population in both pre-cancerous breast lesions and ductal carcinoma in situ, suggesting a potential role in tumorigenesis.[113] Coussens and colleagues have demonstrated that activated B cell paracrine Ig deposition in premalignant lesions is necessary for innate immune cell infiltration, chronic inflammation, and the initiation of de novo carcinogenesis in the K14-HPV16 mouse model of squamous cell carcinoma (SCC).[114] Studies also show that B cell-activated innate immune cells in premalignant lesions promote tumorigenesis by secretion of survival factors, tissue remodeling, and angiogenesis.[115] Furthermore, HIF-1α was found to accumulate throughout PDAC development in both human PDAC tissue samples and the LSL-Kras^{G12D}-Pdx1-Cre GEMM.[116] Deletion of HIF-1α increased PDAC CXCL13 secretion in early pancreatic neoplasia, which recruited TIBs and enhanced PDAC progression. Depletion of B cells reduced PDAC progression, further demonstrating the tumor-promoting role of TIBs.[116]

B cell-mediated pro-tumor immunosuppression is primarily mediated through IL-10-secreting B regulatory (Breg) cells. Studies demonstrate that Bregs are recruited to PDAC tumors by CXCL13-secreting CAFs. These Bregs promote PDAC tumor proliferation through secretion of IL-35 in K-Ras-driven GEMMs of PDAC.[117] These IL-35$^+$ Bregs were also identified as the prominent TIBs in human pancreatic intraepithelial neoplasia and PDAC lesions and correlate with poor prognosis. Furthermore, adoptive transfer of IL-10-secreting Bregs from carcinogen-treated immunocompetent mice were found to restore carcinogen-induced SCC in T and B cell deficient $Tnf^{-/-}Rag2^{-/-}$ mice.[118] Another study showed that Bregs are increased in tongue SCC patient tumors and metastatic lymph nodes; and high Breg infiltrate was associated with poor patient prognosis.[119] Patient-derived tongue SCC cells were found to induce Breg differentiation in co-culture, which were able to induce CD4$^+$ T cell conversion into immunosuppressive Tregs, further implicating the pro-tumor role of TIBs.[119]

A clinical study in BC also revealed that that surgically resected invasive BC tumors were enriched for both immunosuppressive IL-10-secreting Bregs and Tregs compared to fibroadenoma and normal breast tissue and Breg infiltrate increased based on tumor grade, suggesting a correlation with Bregs and malignancy.[120] The study further showed that PD-L1^{hi} human TNBC MDA-MB-231 cells induced the differentiation of CD19$^+$ B cells into Bregs in co-culture, which in turn, induced the differentiation of CD4$^+$ T cells into immunosuppressive FoxP3$^+$ Tregs.[120] Moreover, co-culturing T cells with CD19$^+$ B cells from healthy individuals did not induce Treg differentiation, suggesting that specifically tumor-induced Bregs play a role in maintaining an immunosuppressive TME. Studies by Olkhanud et al further demonstrated that lung metastasis in the 4T1.2 orthotopic TNBC mouse model is dependent on the inhibition of NK cells by Tregs, and the induction of these Tregs were dependent on tumor-induced Bregs.[57,121-123] The study showed that both 4T1 and 4T1.2 tumors and their conditioned medium were able to induce the formation of Bregs both *in vitro* and *in vivo* and that the these cancer-induced Bregs were capable of transforming CD4$^+$ T cells into immunosuppressive FoxP3$^+$ Tregs through Breg-secreted TGF-β in co-culture.[123] Furthermore, both 4T1.2 tumor-bearing T and B cell-deficient NOD/SCID mice or mice treated with either B cell and Treg depleting antibodies did not develop lung metastases. The ability to generate lung metastases in T and B cell deficient NOD/SCID mice was restored upon adoptive transfer of either Tregs or both Tregs and Bregs, but not with Bregs alone.[123] This suggests that these Bregs promote metastasis strictly by inducing Treg formation and do not exhibit a direct tumor-promoting function by themselves.

Studies by Zhang and colleagues further demonstrated the tumor-promoting function Bregs using B-deficient IgM $\mu^{-/-}$ BALB/c mice.[124] The study demonstrated that tumor growth is abrogated, and Treg expansion and function are impaired in B-deficient mice compared to B-proficient Balb/c mice using the allograft EMT6 mouse BC model.[124] Interestingly, adoptive transfer of IL-10⁻ B cells restored Treg function and tumor growth in B cell deficient mice, suggesting that the B cell-mediated Treg promotion is independent of IL-10 secretion. High TIB counts were also found to be associated with increased intra-tumoral Treg proliferation and decreased NK and $CD8^+$ T cell infiltration and anti-tumor function.[124] However, a subsequent study showed that B cell depletion by anti-CD20 antibody treatment failed to fully reject EMT6 tumor growth.[125] Further analysis revealed that while $CD20^+$ B cells were successfully depleted, a small population of $CD20^{low}$ $CD19^+$ B cells remained and Treg populations were maintained.[125] When isolated from primary tumors, these $CD20^{low}$ $CD19^+$ B cells had a greater inhibitory effect on $CD4^+$ T cell function than those isolated from the spleen *in vitro*.[125] This is consistent with the previously reported finding that $CD20^{low}$ Bregs are enriched following anti-CD20 antibody treatment, which enhanced 4T1.2 lung metastasis.[126]

In addition to Bregs, other studies have shown that antibody-secreting PCs may also play a pro-tumor role. One mechanism is through the formation of immune complexes (ICs) in which multiple antigens bind to multiple aggregated antibodies to form their own antigenic molecule.[127]

High circulating IC concentrations have been found in both pre-malignant breast tissue and BC, and correlate with increased tumor growth and poor prognosis.[127,128] Furthermore, a study using a transgenic RIP-Tag2 mouse model of PDAC found that injected non-specific antibodies extravasate and localize at leaky blood vessels in tumor-associated stroma.[128,129] Ig and IC accumulation has been shown to promote ECM degradation, angiogenesis, and accumulation of myeloid cells from Fc receptor binding in the xenograft BC T-47D mouse model.[130] This promoted tumor invasion and metastasis to the lungs and liver in *in vivo* experimental metastasis assays.[130] Utilization of B-deficient IgM $\mu^{-/-}$ mice or B cell depleted mice via anti-IgM antibody administration reduced metastasis formation.[130] Moreover, T and B cell-deficient SCID mice implanted with hybridoma cells producing anti-tumor Igs promoted the growth and metastasis of xenografted human SW620 colon cancer cells compared to non-tumor targeting Igs.[130] Further analysis confirmed that the anti-tumor Ig cohort showed increased tumor stroma IgG deposition, reduced tumor necrosis, increased angiogenesis, and destabilized the ECM near the tumor. These reports are consistent with the study by Coussens and colleagues, which showed that transfer of B cells from HPV16 mice into T and B cell-deficient HVP16 increased IC deposition and chronic inflammation, leading to tumorigenesis in premalignant skin.[114]

PC and pathogenic Ig accumulation have also been reported to promote metastasis outside of the tumor microenvironment as well.[131] Gu and colleagues demonstrated that primary murine TNBC 4T1 and EMT6 orthotopically-implanted tumors induced the accumulation of PCs in tumor-draining lymph nodes as early as one week post implanation.[131] These "tumor-educated" B cells secrete pathogenic IgGs against tumor extracellular HSPA4, which activates HSPA4-binding protein ITGB5 and the src/NF-κB pathway, resulting in tumor expression and secretion of CXCR4 and PGE2, respectively. PGE2 then induces lymphoid stromal cell release of chemokine CXCL12, which binds to tumor-expressed CXCR4 to induce tumor chemotaxis and the formation of lymph node metastases.[131] Taken together, these studies show that Igs can be pathogenic and that tumor-infiltrating PCs and Ig production and deposition in tumors or malignant tissues can promote tumorigenesis, tumor growth, and metastasis.

Despite the studies and evidence covered here regarding the tumor-promoting roles of TIBs, the role of TIBs in cancer and especially metastatic disease remains underexplored compared to other immune cell populations. Furthermore, existing mechanisms of metastasis-promoting B cells are dependent on signaling to other immune or stromal populations and a direct tumor-promoting mechanism only involving B cells and tumor cells remains unknown. However, because of recent findings revealing that TIBs can function in many diverse roles, which can be dependent on spatial localization, further studies are warranted on elucidating the association between B cell localization and function in the context of metastatic disease.

1.3 Systemic Effects of Cancer Metastasis – Cachexia: background, biology

Cachexia Background

Advances in the study of cancer have revealed that the lethality of cancer and metastasis goes beyond the physical and local effects of tumor burden.[132] Tumor cell interactions and signaling with non-tumor cells can trigger the release of soluble factors, metabolites, and exosomes, which systemically alter host metabolism and physiology and contribute to patient mortality.[133] One of the most profoundly lethal systemic effects associated with advanced and metastatic cancer patients is cachexia, derived from the Greek lexicon: kakos" and "hexis" - meaning bad and condition, respectively.[134-136] The term cancer cachexia was first coined by English ophthalmologist John Zachariah Laurence in 1858 in referring to the body wasting syndrome exhibited by cancer patients.[134] Although the formal definition of cachexia has varied since, an international consensus in 2011 defined cancer cachexia as "a multifactorial syndrome defined by an ongoing loss of skeletal muscle mass (with or without loss of fat mass) that cannot be fully reserved by conventional nutritional support and leads to progressive functional impairment".[137] The consensus of clinical diagnosis criteria for cancer cachexia was defined as a greater than 5% loss of body weight or a greater than 2% loss of body weight in patients that already exhibit weight loss or sarcopenia.[137] Furthermore, cachexia was determined to be a progressive disease with multiple stages – pre-cachexia, cachexia, and refractory cachexia - and can be classified into each by the severity of body protein and weight loss.[137]

The incidence of cachexia varies by cancer type, with the highest incidence of 87% among PDAC and gastric cancer patients and lower incidences of around 40% in BC, sarcomas, and leukemias.[136] However, because obesity and weight gain is a risk factor for BC patients, cachexia diagnoses by weight loss alone may not accurately detect cachexia in many patients.[135,138,139] Regardless of cancer type, cachexia presents as a severe and debilitating body and muscle wasting syndrome characterized by dysregulated metabolism and systemic inflammation.[134,135,137] The development of cachexia significantly reduces patient survival and is responsible for approximately 20% of all cancer-related mortality and up to 80% of all advanced PDAC-associated mortality.[140-142] The primary cause of death from cachexia stems from the loss of muscle mass and function, the proper function of which are necessary for vital functions such as breathing, locomotion, ingestion of food, and pumping blood.[143] Additionally, not only can chemotherapy exacerbate or worsen cachexia symptoms by inducing weight loss, inflammation, fatigue, and release of cachexia-promoting cytokines, but cachectic patients also exhibit a decreased tolerance to chemotherapeutic agents, thus limiting treatment options.[144,145]

Cachexia Biology

It is important to recognize that weight loss from cachexia is distinct from age-related sarcopenia, anorexia/starvation, malabsorption, and hyperthyroidism.[134,135,137] The distinction between weight loss in cancer cachexia and anorexia or sarcopenia is that weight loss from cachexia presents with a reduction in muscle mass caused by increase in resting energy expenditure, systemic inflammation, is independent of adipose tissue loss, and a decrease in muscle-protein synthesis coupled with an increase in energy and protein catabolism mediated by ubiquitin-proteosome degradation and autophagy pathways.[133,141,146] Importantly, weight loss in cachectic patients cannot be reversed by nutritional support. Conversely, weight loss in anorexia or sarcopenia is reversible with nutritional support, and presents without inflammation, increase in protein catabolism, or increases in resting energy expenditure.[147,148]

Metastasis and cachexia are intricately linked, as the aberrant metabolic and systemic reprogramming of host physiology necessary for metastasis ultimately culminates to the development of cachexia at the systemic level.[149] Studies in mouse models of PDAC have shown that 1) complete surgical resection of the tumor can reverse cachexia and 2) experimental metastasis assays can induce cachexia in the absence of a primary tumor.[150] These confirm that the induction and maintenance of cachexia is requires either a primary tumor or metastatic colonies. Furthermore, studies using parabiotic experiments to exchange blood flow between sarcoma tumor-bearing (Tb) and non tumor-bearing (nTb) rats revealed that nTb parabiotic rats also developed cachexia, indicating that a Tb host contains humoral cachexia-promoting circulating factors.[151,152] Following studies utilizing both primary tumor and experimental metastasis mouse models of cachexia have revealed that cachexia-promoting factors are highly diverse and can originate from either tumor cells, non-tumor cells within the TME, or distant organs and these factors can either interact with muscle cells directly or reprogram the metabolism of other organs and tissues to induce muscle atrophy.[133,152,153]

Muscle mass loss in cachexia is internally mediated by increased muscle protein catabolism and reduced muscle protein synthesis, as cancer cells reprogram the host metabolism to increase their own nutrient uptake and proliferation.[133,153] Cachexia muscle protein catabolism is driven by increased activity of muscle ubiquitin-proteosome degradation pathways, which is mediated by transcriptional upregulation of muscle atrophy-related E3 ubiquitin ligases, such as muscle-specific RING finger protein 1 (MURF1 or TRIM63), muscle atrophy F-box protein (MAFBX or FBXO32), FBXO31, and FBXO30 (MUSA1).[133,153]

Tumor and non-tumor cells in the TME secrete a multitude of soluble factors into circulation, including proinflammatory cytokines, such as TNF-α, IL-1β, IL-6, and IL-8, and immunosuppressive cytokines, such as TGF-β.[133,153] The TGF-β family member, myostatin, is a known negative regulator of muscle growth and functions by activating muscle smad-2 to inhibit downstream proliferation-promoting Akt and mTORC1 pathways.[154] TNF-α can activate downstream the NF-κB pathway in muscle cells to drive 1) upregulation of muscle atrophy-related E3 ubiquitin ligases to mediate muscle protein breakdown and 2) the posttranscriptional suppression of MyoD mRNA, which is responsible for muscle-cell differentiation.[155,156] The proinflammatory cytokines, TNF-α, IL-1β, IL-6, and IL-8, also induce fatty acid oxidation in muscles cells, resulting in high levels of oxidative stress, which activates the p38-MAPK stress response pathway to impair myotube growth.[157]

Similarly, extracellular vesicles (EVs) released from malignant cells can contain heat shock proteins HSP70 and HSP90 can activate toll-like receptor 4 (TLR4) on muscle cells, which also activates the p38-MAPK pathway.[158] Tumor-derived EVs containing microRNA-21 have also been shown to activate toll-like receptor 7 (TLR7) on myoblasts to promote myoblast apoptosis.[159]

Circulating factors can also indirectly mediate cachexia by altering the metabolism of other organs to increase resting energy expenditure. Tumor-derived factors, such as IL-6 and parathyroid hormone-related protein, can induce chronic inflammation within white adipose tissue (WAT).[160] This increases the expression of uncoupling protein 1 (UCP1) in WAT, which uncouples ATP synthesis and oxidative respiration to increase thermogenesis and the browning of WAT into beige adipose tissue.[160] Beige adipose tissue exhibits increased lipolysis compared to WAT, which ultimately increases host resting energy expenditure and has been demonstrated in multiple mouse models of PDAC, lung, CRC, and hepatic cancer.[160] Furthermore, tumor-derived IL-6 activates STAT3 in liver hepatocytes and lung tissue to drive production of pro-inflammatory acute phase response (APR) proteins, resulting in the massive synthesis of plasma proteins.[152,153] To meet this high demand for amino acids needed for APR-induced protein synthesis, skeletal muscle proteins are catabolized, leading to muscle atrophy.[153] These APR proteins also include ECM components, such as fibronectin and fibrinogen, the synthesis of which can induced by other tumor-derived factors (e.g. TNF-α, TGF-β and VEGFA), resulting in inflammation and fibrosis of liver and lung microenvironments that primes the organs for metastatic colonization.[153] Taken together, these examples demonstrate that tumor-derived factors can alter the metabolism of distant organs to drive both cachexia and metastasis. Moreover, because metastatic tumor cells also secrete tumor-derived factors and modulate their host organs, the progression of cancer into metastatic disease further accelerates the development and exacerbation of muscle atrophy and cachexia.

However, despite the elucidation of many mechanisms that mediate cancer cachexia and over a hundred clinical trials targeting various mediators of cachexia, there currently remains no approved or effective treatments for cachexia in cancer patients.[161] The high prevalence, lethality, and lack of treatment for cachexia highlights a dire need for the discovery of targetable novel mediators for cancer cachexia and the *in vivo* targeting of these mediators in preclinical models. Furthermore, because of how cancer metastasis and cachexia are intricately linked in both mechanism and patient prognosis, these treatment targets should focus on mediators of cachexia in the context of metastatic disease.

Chapter 2: Upregulation of ZIP14 and elevated Zinc levels in pancreatic cancer cachexia

2.1 Zinc and ZIP14: biological function and effects on cancer cachexia

Biological function

Zinc (Zn^{2+}) is trace metal that plays a vital role in many biological processes. About 10% of all human proteins binds to Zn^{2+} and Zn^{2+} functions as a cofactor for more than 300 enzymes and 2000 transcription factors.[162] However, serum and intracellular zinc concentrations must be strictly regulated, as excess zinc is toxic and zinc deficiency impairs host growth, immune response, metabolism, and can result in hypogonadism.[162] Adult humans typically contain a total of 2-3g of zinc, 57% and 29% of which are located within skeletal muscle and bone, respectively.[163] Extracellular zinc is found in serum, with 75-85% of serum zinc being bound to albumin.[164] However, unlike other nutrients, humans do not have a reserve or storage organ for zinc. Therefore, zinc levels must be consistently replenished by nutritional intake and a carefully regulated homeostasis between extracellular and intracellular zinc levels must be maintained.[165] In mammals, intra and extracellular zinc concentrations are regulated by two families of zinc transporters, the SLC30 (ZnT) exporter and SLC39 (ZIP) importer families, which decrease and increase intracellular zinc, respectively.[162] The ZIP family encompasses 14 members: SLC39A1-SLC39A14 (ZIP1-ZIP14) and are widely expressed in different tissues and cell types.

Effects on cancer cachexia

Clinical studies have observed that serum zinc concentrations are reduced in multiple types of cancers, including those with high incidences of cachexia, such as PDAC, lung cancer, and CRC.[166-168] In 2010, decreased serum zinc and aberrant systemic zinc redistribution were hypothesized to play a role in the development of cachexia, as 1) APR and dysregulated immune response often presented in cachectic patients and 2) cachectic patients and zinc deficient patients both exhibit similar impaired growth, immune response, and metabolic functions.[165] Because humans lack a functional zinc reserve, decreased serum zinc would suggest that extracellular zinc has been aberrantly distributed into specific tissues. Studies utilizing preclinical mouse models of fibrosarcoma and CRC have shown that tumor-bearing cachectic muscles exhibit significantly elevated zinc concentrations, suggesting that extracellular zinc is aberrantly imported into cachectic muscles.[169,170] However, the link between aberrant muscle zinc concentration, muscle wasting and cachexia, and cancer and metastasis remained largely unknown, until recent findings from our laboratory.

Based on the these correlations, Acharyya et al investigated the mechanisms involving metastasis and zinc homeostasis in cachectic muscles using murine metastatic allograft models, 4T1 (TNBC), C26m2 (CRC), and KP1 (lung cancer), a xenograft PC9-Brm3 (lung cancer) model, and the $K\text{-}ras^{LSL\text{-}G12D/+}$, $p53^{fl/fl}$, $Pten^{fl/fl}$, $Lkb1^{fl/fl}$ (lung cancer) GEMM.[171] Allograft and xenograft models had their primary tumors surgically resected 2-3 weeks post-implantation to eliminate the effects and complications of a primary tumor, leaving only distant metastases. Therefore, these resected models specifically represent the interactions and effects between metastasis and cachexia. Metastasis was detected and confirmed by bioluminescent imaging using the *in vivo* imaging system (IVIS) and by histological analysis of metastatic organs. The development of cachexia was confirmed by 1) significant decrease in body mass throughout tumor progression, 2) morphometric analysis of tibialis anterior (TA) muscles, which revealed that Tb mouse muscle fiber cross-sectional area (CSA) was reduced compared to nTb mice, and 3) amplified transcription of muscle atrophy-related E3 ubiquitin ligases (*Murf1*, *Mafbx*, *Fbxo31*, and *Musa1*) in TA, diaphragm (DIA), extensor digitorum longus (EDL), soleus, gastrocnemius (GAST) quadriceps (QUAD), and cardiac muscles.[171]

The *Zip14* gene was found to be transcriptionally upregulated, even compared to other *Zip* family genes, by transcriptomic RNA-sequencing (RNA-seq) analysis of cachectic TA, DIA, EDL, GAST, QUAD, and cardiac muscles from 4T1, C27m2, PC9-Brm3, and *K-ras*$^{LSL-G12D/+}$, *p53*$^{fl/fl}$, *Pten*$^{fl/fl}$, *Lkb1*$^{fl/fl}$ models compared to those of healthy nTb mice.[171] This suggests that *Zip14* expression is correlated with the expression of muscle atrophy-associated E3 ubiquitin ligases and cachexia development in multiple muscles groups associated with vital functions. Furthermore, *Zip14* was not upregulated in the muscles of a non-metastatic GEMM of lung cancer and a non-cachectic metastatic allograft lung cancer model, which suggests that the muscle upregulation of *Zip14* is specific to the context of metastasis-induced cachexia.[171] These results were validated by immunohistochemical staining and analysis of ZIP14 expression in non-cachectic and cachectic muscle samples from human cancer patients. Blinded pathological analysis revealed high ZIP14-specific staining in the atrophic muscle fibers 19 out of 43 cachectic cancer patients and 8 of out of 53 non-cachectic patients, with low or no signal in non-atrophic muscle fibers.[171] This confirms that ZIP14 protein expression is elevated in atrophic muscles of advanced cancer patients.

The study revealed that induction of *Zip14* expression during tumor progression and cachexia development was mediated by tumor-derived TGF-β and TNF-α cytokines though *in vitro* and *in vivo* functional assays. Treatment of human primary muscle cells and murine C2C12 myoblasts with either recombinant TGF-β or TNF-α induced *Zip14* expression while inhibition of respective downstream SMAD and NF-κB pathways with respective inhibitors blocked *Zip14* expression.[171] Furthermore, elevated serum and TME levels of TGF-β and TNF-α have been reported in both human patients and mouse models and treatment of 4T1 and C26m2 mouse models with either TGF-β or TNF-α neutralizing antibodies significantly reduced muscle expression of *Zip14*.[171]

To determine the role of *Zip14* expression in metastasis-induced cachexia, Acharyya et al generated *Zip14* germline deletion and muscle-specific conditional knockdown of *Zip14* mouse models. These displayed no defect in tumor growth or metastasis compared to wild-type control, but both germline *Zip14*-null and muscle-specific *Zip14* knockdown models demonstrated a significant rescue of body weight loss and muscle atrophy compared to wild-type controls.[171] These results suggest that muscle *Zip14* expression is required for the development of metastasis-induced cachexia.

Furthermore, the study revealed that ZIP14 mediates metastasis-induced cachexia through its canonical function as a zinc importer. Inductively coupled-plasma mass spectrometry (ICP-MS) confirmed an increased in muscle-zinc concentrations and a concomitant reduction in serum zinc concentrations in cachectic 4T1 and C26m2 mouse models. Conversely, tumor-bearing germline *Zip14*-null mice exhibited no difference in muscle-zinc levels compared to non tumor-bearing mice. Furthermore, zinc supplementation exacerbated body weight loss and muscle atrophy in wild-type, but not *Zip14*-null mice without any alterations in tumor growth in either model. Subsequent *in vitro* experiments revealed that accumulation of zinc in *Zip14*-expressing myoblasts and myotubules resulted in loss of *MyoD* and *Mef2c* expression, which resulted in the blockade of myotube differentiation, and loss of myosin heavy chain (MyHC), respectively.[171] Taken together, these findings demonstrate that metastatic cancer-secreted TGF-β and TNF-α induce aberrant muscle expression of *Zip14*, which increases intracellular zinc that leads to muscle atrophy and the development of cachexia in mouse models of lung, breast, and lung cancer.

2.2 Generation and validation of experimental metastasis mouse models of pancreatic adenocarcinoma cachexia

PDAC patients exhibit one of the highest mortality rates among cancers, with an overall five-year survival rate of 9% that drops to 2% for metastatic patients.[172,173] A major factor contributing to its lethality is that PDAC has the highest incidence of cachexia among cancers, with approximately 87% of diagnosed patients developing cachexia over the course of disease progression.[136] Furthermore, most PDAC patients are diagnosed when the cancer has already progressed to locally advanced stage III or stage IV metastatic disease, which limits opportunities for surgical resection, which is the only curative option for PDAC.[174-177] The high incidence of cachexia and its significant impact on patient mortality underscores the importance of elucidating the mechanisms of PDAC-induced cachexia to uncover potential targets for therapeutic intervention.

To determine the mechanisms mediating PDAC-induced cachexia, we generated two experimental metastasis models of PDAC that utilize the murine PDAC cell lines: Pan02 and FC1242. These cell lines were selected to model metastatic human PDAC based on the following criteria: 1) the ability of metastasize and induce cachexia, and 2) different mutational landscapes to rule out cell line- or mutation- specific effects. The Pan02 cell line is a metastatic $SMAD4^{null}$ murine PDAC cell line derived from a 3-methylcholanthrene carcinogen-induced primary pancreatic tumor that developed in a C57BL/6 background mouse.[178,179] The FC1242 cell line was derived from a primary pancreatic tumor that developed in a $LSL\text{-}Kras^{G12D}$; $LSL\text{-}Trp53^{R172H}$; $Pdx1\text{-}Cre$ GEMM with a C57BL/6 background.[178] We generated experimental metastasis models through intracardiac injection of 1×10^5 murine Pan02 and FC1242 into arterial circulation in male 8- to 9- week old athymic nude and syngeneic C57BL/6 mice, respectively (Figure 2-1A). The Pan02 and FC1242 experimental metastasis models gradually developed metastasis and cachexia, which were confirmed by histological analysis and measurements of weight loss, hind-limb grip strength, muscle fiber CSA, and muscle expression of muscle atrophy-associated E3 ubiquitin ligases (Figure 2-1B-H). Both Pan02 and FC1242 experimental metastasis models exhibit a significant loss in body weight and reduction of hind limb functional grip strength by endpoint, along with the development of lung and liver metastases, when compared to age-matched healthy control mice (Figure 2-1B-E). The loss of muscle function demonstrated by reduction of hind limb grip strength was found to be associated with a decrease in muscle fiber size, which was quantified by morphometric analysis of muscle fiber CSA (Figure 2-1F, G). Pan02 and FC1242 experimental metastasis model GAST muscles displayed histological features of muscle atrophy, reduced size, and contained a lower percentage of muscle fibers with larger CSA and a higher percentage of muscle fibers with smaller CSA when compared to healthy control mice (Figure 2-1F, G). Furthermore, cachectic GAST muscles from Pan02 and FC1242 experimental metastasis models exhibited elevated expression of *Murf1*, *Mafbx*, *Fbxo31*, and *Musa1* muscle atrophy-associated E3 ubiquitin ligases (Figure 2-1H) compared to healthy control mice. Taken together, these results suggest that the Pan02 and FC1242 PDAC experimental metastasis models develop metastatic disease along with the concomitant development of cachexia.

A
Intra-cardiac
Injection
of PDAC
cell lines
Metastasis and cachexia

B
Pan02 model
FC1242 model
Body weight change (%)
Con
Tb
120
100
80
60
p = 0.0089
110
100
90
80
p = 0.01
0 1 2 3 4
Time (weeks)

C
Con
Tb
Pan02 model
% grip strength
n.s.   p = 0.0008
120
100
80
60
40
20
0
Initial Final Initial Final
FC1242 model
% grip strength
n.s.   p < 0.0001
120
100
80
60
40
20
0
Initial Final Initial Final
Con   Tb

D
Liver
FC1242 model
Con
Tb

E
Lung
Pan02 model   FC1242 model
Con
Tb

F
Gastrocnemius muscle
Pan02 model   FC1242 model
Con
Tb

G
Gastrocnemius muscle
Con
Tb
Pan02 model
Percentage of fibers (%)
100
75
50
25
0
p = 0.026   p = 0.036   n.s.   p = 0.647
0-500   501-1000   1001-2000   2001-3000
FC1242 model
100
75
50
25
0
p = 0.001   p = 0.023   p = 0.019   p = 0.028
0-500   501-1000   1001-2000   2001-3000
Fiber cross section area (µm²)

H
Gastrocnemius muscle
Trim63   Fbxo32   Fbxo31   Fbxo30
Con
Tb
Pan02 model
Relative mRNA expression
p = 0.0017   p = 0.0015   p < 0.0001   p = 0.0410
Con Tb   Con Tb   Con Tb   Con Tb
FC1242 model
p = 0.0007   p = 0.0226   p = 0.0261   p = 0.0214
Con Tb   Con Tb   Con Tb   Con Tb

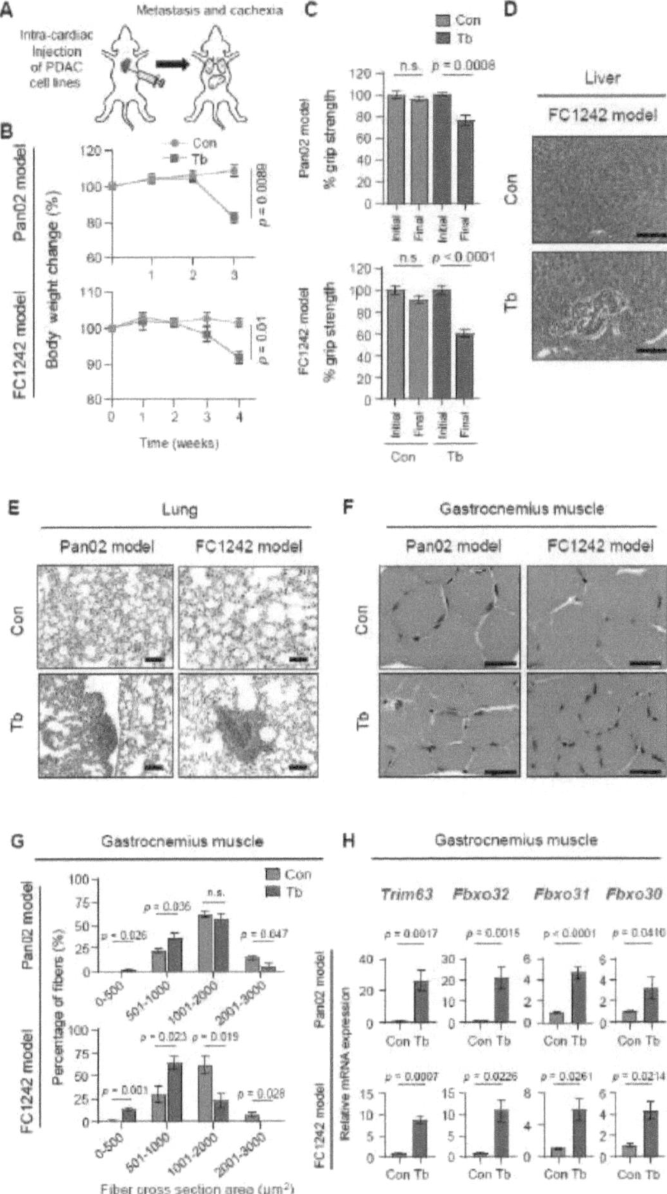

43

Figure 2-1: Cachexia development in Pan02 and FC1242 experimental metastasis models of pancreatic ductal adenocarcinoma (PDAC)

(**A**) Schematic depicting the intra-cardiac injection of 1 x 10^5 Pan02 or FC1242 cells into the arterial circulation of mice and subsequent development of metastasis. (**B**) Body weight measurements of Pan02 and FC1242 experimental metastasis models (Tb, blue lines) compared to non tumor-bearing control mice (Con, gray lines). (**C**) Measurements of hind-limb grip strength in Pan02 and FC1242 experimental metastasis models (Tb, blue bars) compared to control (Con, gray bars) mice before tumor-cell injection (initial) and at endpoint (final). Data is normalized to the mean of initial values of each group. (**D**) Representative images of hematoxylin and eosin- (H&E) stained liver tissue sections from the FC1242 experimental metastasis model compared to control mice. Scale bars represent 100 μm. (**E**) Representative images of H&E-stained lung tissue sections from Pan02 and FC1242 experimental metastasis models compared to control mice. Scale bars represent 100 μm. (**F**) Representative images of H&E-stained gastrocnemius muscle cross-sections from Pan02 and FC1242 experimental metastasis models compared to control mice. Scale bars represent 25 μm. (**G**) Quantitation of gastrocnemius muscle fiber cross-sectional area (CSA) from Pan02 and FC1242 experimental metastasis models compared to control mice. Morphometric analysis is shown as the distribution frequency of muscle fibers stratified by CSA ranges. (**H**) Results from real-time quantitative reverse transcription PCR (RT-qPCR) analysis of muscle atrophy markers *Trim63* (*Murf1*), *Fbxo32* (*Mafbx*), *Fbxo31*, and *Fbxo30* (*Musa1*) in the gastrocnemius muscles from Pan02 (top) and FC1242 (bottom) experimental metastasis models compared to control mice. $n = 3$–5 mice/group. Data are expressed as mean $\pm$ standard error of the mean (SEM). *p*-values were determined by the two-tailed, unpaired Student's t-test. n.s., Not significant; Con, control; Tb, tumor-bearing.

<u>**2.3 Cachectic gastrocnemius muscles exhibit upregulated ZIP14 expression and elevated intramuscular zinc concentration in Pan02 and FC1242 experimental metastasis models of pancreatic adenocarcinoma**</u>

Continuing our studies that demonstrated that muscle upregulation of *Zip14* expression and elevated intramuscular zinc concentration mediate cachexia in metastatic mouse models of colon, breast, and lung cancer,[171] we analyzed the role of the *Zip14*-zinc axis in the cachectic muscles from Pan02 and FC1242 experimental metastasis models. Quantitative RT-qPCR and immunoblot analysis revealed that the cachectic GAST muscles of Pan02 and FC1242 experimental metastasis models had significantly upregulated expression and protein levels of *Zip14* when compared to nTb control mice (Figure 2-2A, B). These results are consistent with our previous findings.[171]

Because ZIP14 is a broad-spectrum importer for not only zinc, but iron (Fe^{2+}) and manganese (Mn^{2+}) as well, we analyzed the intramuscular levels of these metal ions along with copper (Cu^{2+}) as a negative control in GAST muscles by ICP-MS.[180] The results revealed that zinc ion levels were elevated in the cachectic GAST muscles of Pan02 and FC1242 experimental models compared to control mice (Figure 2-2C). A small increase manganese levels was detected in the Pan02, but not the FC1242, experimental metastasis model and there were no significant alterations in manganese or copper levels in either model (Figure 2-2C). This suggests that upregulated *Zip14* in the cachectic GAST muscles functions primarily in its zinc import role. Concomitant with elevated *Zip14* expression and intramuscular zinc concentration, cachectic GAST muscles also exhibited significantly upregulated expression of zinc-inducible and zinc-binding metallothionein (*Mt*) proteins 1 (*Mt1*) and 2 (*Mt2*) (Figure 2-2D).[181,182] Mt proteins contain cysteine-rich metal-binding domains and are markers for aberrantly elevated intracellular zinc concentrations.[181,182] Taken together, these findings demonstrate that cachectic muscles of Pan02 and FC1242 experimental metastasis models harbor concomitant elevated *Zip14* expression, aberrant elevated intramuscular zinc levels, and elevated *Mt*1 and *Mt2* expression.

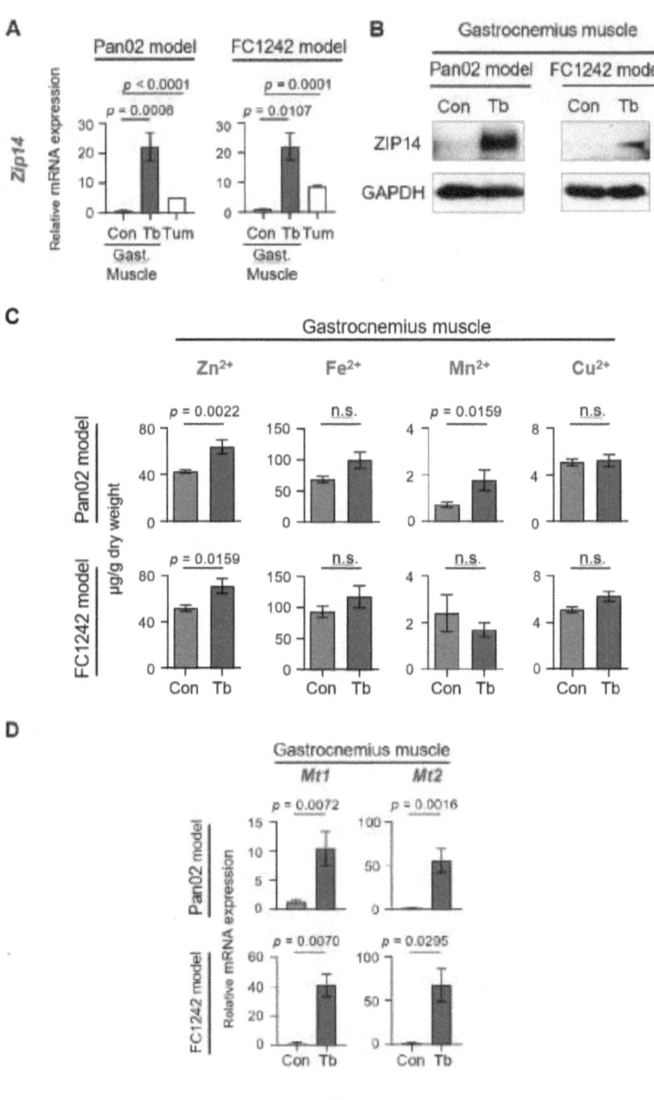

Figure 2-2: Zip14 is induced and associated with elevated zinc levels in the cachectic muscles of experimental metastasis models of pancreatic adenocarcinoma (PDAC)

(**A**) Results from RT-qPCR analysis of *Zip14* expression in the gastrocnemius (Gast.) muscles from Pan02 (left) and FC1242 (right) experimental metastasis models (Tb, blue bars) compared to control mice (Con, gray bars) and Pan02 and FC1242 cell lines (Tum, white bars). (**B**) Immunoblot analysis probing for ZIP14 in gastrocnemius (Gast.) muscle-cell lysate from Pan02 (left) and FC1242 (right) experimental metastasis models compared to control mice. GAPDH was used as an internal control. Data is representative of three independent experiments. (**C**) Results from metal ion analysis of zinc (Zn^{2+}), iron (Fe^{2+}), manganese (Mn^{2+}), and copper (Cu^{2+}) in gastrocnemius muscles from Pan02 (top) and FC1242 (bottom) experimental metastasis models compared to control mice at endpoint. Data is expresed as micrograms (mg) of metal ions per gram (g) of muscle dry weight. (**D**) Results from RT-qPCR analysis of *Mt1* and *Mt2* expression in the gastrocnemius muscles from Pan02 (top) and FC1242 (bottom) experimental metastasis models (Tb, blue bars) compared to control mice (Con, gray bars) at endpoint. $n = 3–5$ mice/group. Data are represented as the mean $\pm$ SEM. *p*-values for RT-qPCR analysis were determined by using the two-tailed, unpaired Student's *t*-test. *p*-values for metal ion analysis were determined by using the Mann–Whitney test. Con, control; Tb, Tumor-bearing; Tum, tumor cell lines; Gast., Gastrocnemius muscle.

2.4 Clinical validation of elevated ZIP14 expression in cachectic pectoralis muscles from advanced pancreatic adenocarcinoma patients

To clinically validate our experimental findings that associate the *Zip14*-zinc axis with metastatic PDAC-induced cachexia, we performed immunohistochemical staining and analysis of

ZIP14 expression in pectoralis muscle sections from human cachectic and non-cachectic advanced PDAC patients (Figure 2-3A, B). Blinded pathological analysis revealed significantly more ZIP14-positive staining in the atrophic pectoralis muscle fibers from cachectic PDAC patients (75%) compared to the muscle fibers of non-cachectic PDAC patients (42.9%) (Figure 2-3B). Furthermore, ZIP14-positive staining was restricted to and observed specifically in the atrophic muscle fibers from cachectic PDAC patients (Figure 2-4A). These results are consistent with our experimental results that show that cachectic muscles from Pan02 and FC1242 experimental metastasis models exhibit elevated *Zip14* expression compared to control mice (Figures 2-1 and 2-2).

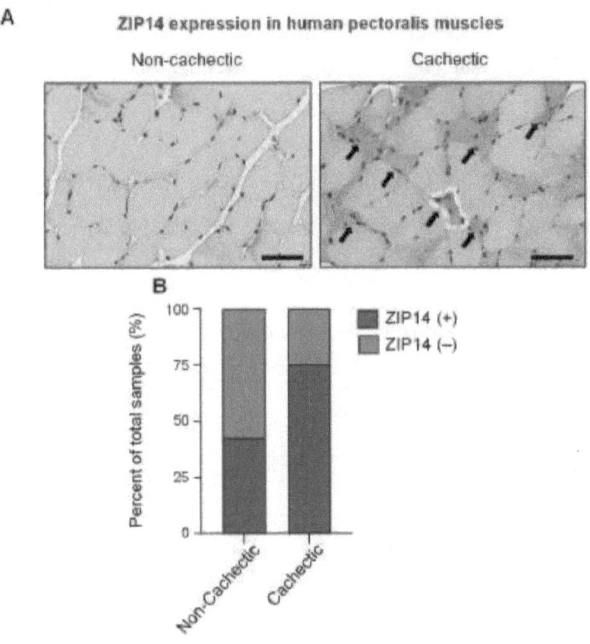

Figure 2-3: Clinical validation of elevated ZIP14 expression in cachectic pectoralis muscles from patients with metastatic pancreatic adenocarcinoma (PDAC)

(**A**) Representative images of human pectoralis muscle cross-sections from non-cachectic (left, *n* = 7) and cachectic (right, *n* = 12) PDAC patients immunostained with antibodies against human ZIP14. A representative atrophic fiber is marked by the yellow dotted line. Additional atrophic fibers in the field of view are marked with black arrows. Scale bars represent 50 μm. (**B**) Blinded pathological analysis and scoring of ZIP14-stained pectoralis muscle sections from human non-cachectic and cachectic PDAC patients as ZIP14-positive (ZIP14 (+), blue bars) or ZIP14-negative (ZIP14 (-), gray bars). Data are shown as a percentage of total samples. The *p*-value was calculated using Pearson's chi-square test on scored sample counts (*p* = 0.0005).

2.5 *Zip14* expression is upregulated in the cachectic diaphragm muscles of Pan02 and FC1242 experimental metastasis models and cachectic human pancreatic adenocarcinoma patients

To confirm the systemic upregulation *Zip14* in skeletal muscles during the development of cachexia, we analyzed DIA muscles for the upregulation of muscle atrophy markers, *Zip14*, and *Mt* expression in the Pan02 and FC1242 experimental metastasis models. DIA muscles are skeletal muscles that are intricately and functionally linked to respiration and compromised DIA muscle function can result in respiratory failure and poor survival in cachectic cancer patients.[183,184] Histological analysis of H&E-stained DIA muscle sections from Pan02 and FC1242 experimental metastasis models revealed significant reduction in muscle fiber size when compared to control mice (Figure 2-4A). The presence of muscle atrophy was further confirmed by RT-qPCR, which revealed that the DIA muscles from Pan02 and FC1242 experimental metastasis models exhibited significant upregulated expression of *Murf1*, *Mafbx*, *Fbxo31*, and *Musa1* muscle atrophy-associated E3 ubiquitin ligases compared to control mice (Figure 2-4B). Furthermore, similar to GAST muscles, *Zip14* and zinc-inducible *Mt1* and *Mt2* expression were found to be significantly upregulated in the cachectic DIA muscles of Pan02 and FC1242 experimental metastasis models compared to control mice (Figure 2-4C).

To clinically validate these experimental findings, we performed immunohistochemical staining and analysis of ZIP14 expression in DIA muscle sections from human cachectic and non-cachectic advanced PDAC patients (Figure 2-4D). Blinded pathological analysis revealed significantly more ZIP14-positive staining in the atrophic DIA muscle fibers from cachectic PDAC patients (100%) compared to the muscle fibers of non-cachectic PDAC patients (23.19%) (Figure 2-4E). Taken together, the elevated expression of muscle atrophy-associated E3 ubiquitin ligases, *Zip14* and *Mt1* and *Mt2* in both GAST and DIA muscles of Pan02 and FC1242 experimental metastasis models, along with strong ZIP14-positive staining in both GAST and DIA muscles of cachectic advanced PDAC patients suggests that the aberrant *Zip14*-zinc axis is systemically present in skeletal muscles during the development PDAC-induced cachexia.

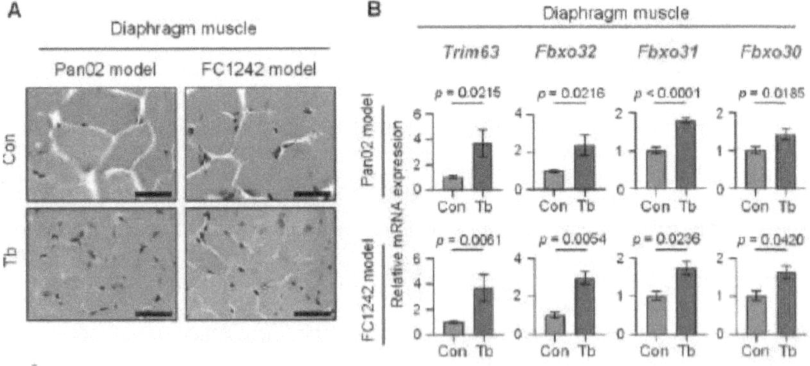

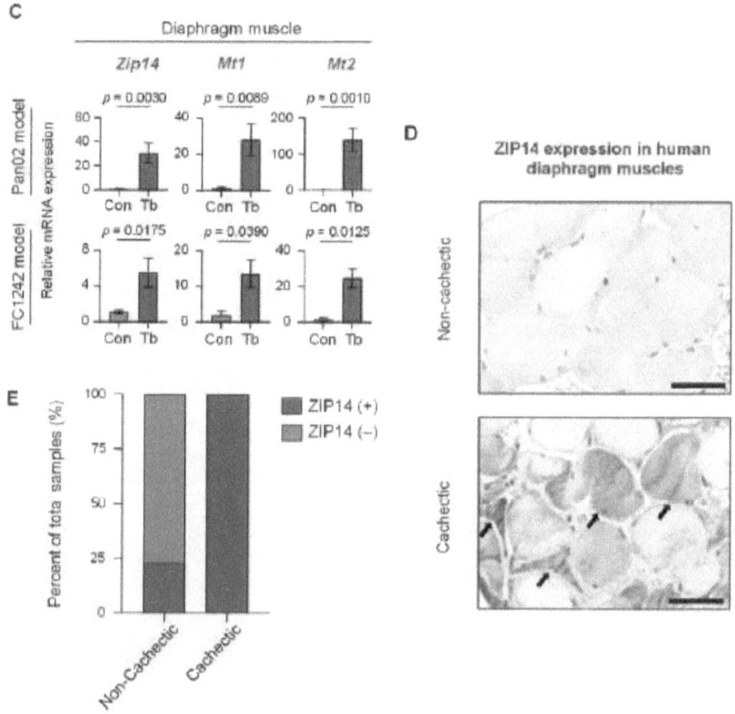

Figure 2-4. ZIP14 expression in diaphragm muscles from pancreatic adenocarcinoma (PDAC) experimental metastasis mouse models and human patients

(A) Representative images of diaphragm muscle cross-sections stained with H&E from Pan02 and FC1242 experimental metastasis mice compared to control mice. Scale bars represent 25 μm. (B) Results from RT-qPCR analysis of *Trim63* (*Murf1*), *Fbxo32* (*Mafbx*), *Fbxo31*, and *Fbxo30* (*Musa1*) in the diaphragm muscles from Pan02 (top) and FC1242 (bottom) experimental metastasis models (Tb, blue bars) compared to control mice (Con, gray bars). (C) Results from RT-qPCR analysis of *Zip14*, *Mt1*, and *Mt2* in the diaphragm muscles from Pan02 (top) and

FC1242 (bottom) experimental metastasis models compared to control mice. (**D**) Representative images human diaphragm muscle cross-sections immunostained with antibodies against human ZIP14 from non-cachectic (top, $n = 13$) and cachectic (bottom, $n = 10$) advanced PDAC patients. A representative atrophic fiber is marked by the yellow dotted line. Additional atrophic fibers visualized in the field are marked with arrows. Scale bars represent 25 μm. (**E**) Blinded scoring of ZIP14-stained human diaphragm muscle sections as ZIP14-positive (ZIP14 (+), blue bars) or ZIP14-negative (ZIP14 (-), gray bars) from non-cachectic and cachectic advanced PDAC patients. $n = 3$–6 mice/group. Data for RT-qPCR analysis are represented as the mean $\pm$ SEM. Data for ZIP14 pathological scoring are shown as a percentage of total samples. *p*-values for RT-qPCR analysis were determined using the two-tailed, unpaired Student's *t*-test. *p*-values for ZIP14 pathological scoring were determined using the Pearson's chi-square test ($p < 0.0001$). Con: Control; Tb: Tumor-bearing.

2.6 Discussion

Analogous to our lab's previous work on metastatic BC-, CRC-, and lung cancer-induced cachexia,[185] here, we show that aberrant muscle-cell upregulation of the zinc importer, *Zip14*, correlates with 1) increased intramuscular zinc levels, 2) elevated zinc-inducible *Mt* expression, and 3) elevated expression of muscle atrophy-associated E3 ubiquitin ligases in the cachectic GAST and DIA muscles from two independent experimental metastasis models of PDAC. Furthermore, we show that pectoralis and DIA muscles from cachectic human advanced PDAC patients have exhibit elevated ZIP14 expression when compared to non-cachectic patients. Future studies are warranted to determine at what timepoint during PDAC progression and cachexia development is *Zip14* expression induced in muscle cells and to determine and subsequently validate if a clinical association exists between patient PDAC stage and ZIP14 induction in patient muscle cells. Our previous work had also revealed that tumor-associated TNF-α and TGF-β cytokines can upregulate ZIP14 expression in muscle cells and myoblasts.[171] It is known that TNF-α and TGF-β are present in the conditioned media of PDAC cell lines and in the serum of PDAC patients.[178,186-189] Therefore, further *in vivo* studies are needed to determine if pharmacologic blockade of either TNF-α or TGF-β signaling in muscle cells can reduce *Zip14* expression and inhibit or slow the development of PDAC-induced cachexia. The identification of TNF-α, TGF-β, and other potential factors that mediate muscle upregulation of ZIP14 in PDAC can have critical clinical implications as they can be used as 1) biomarkers to determine cachexia development and 2) potential druggable targets to manage cachexia development in PDAC patients.

In addition to targeting mediators of *Zip14* expression, directly targeting and inhibiting ZIP14 function or metal chelation therapy to reduce intramuscular zinc levels could be tested as a therapeutic strategy to treat PDAC-induced cachexia. A recent study had demonstrated that treatment of human PDAC cell lines with TPEN (N, N, N'',N'-Tetrakis (2-pyridylmethyl)-ethylenediamine), a membrane-permeable intracellular zinc chelator, induced tumor cell death by reducing GSH levels, increasing oxidative stress, and promoting mitochondrial dysfunction.[190] Furthermore, zinc chelator-induced tumor cell death has also been reported in leukemia, BC, osteosarcoma, and prostate cancer cell lines *in vitro*, although *in vivo* zinc chelation assays in PDAC mouse models have yet to be performed.[191-196] Taken together, our previous studies,[185] and these current findings provide a strong rationale for testing the efficacy of ZIP14 inhibition and zinc chelation strategies in PDAC-induced cachexia.

Chapter 3: Aberrant Zip14 expression in muscle is associated with cachexia in a Bard1-deficient mouse model of triple-negative breast cancer

<u>**3.1 Cachexia and *BRCA*-mutant breast cancer**</u>

Until recently, BC patients have been associated with lower incidences of cachexia.[136] However, computed tomography (CT) analysis of body composition of BC patients have revealed that cachexia-associated weight loss and muscle wasting is often masked by BC-associated obesity and gain of excess adipose tissue.[197-200] Because cachexia is typically diagnosed using loss of body weight, the prevalence of cachexia in BC patients is often underdiagnosed in the clinic. Building upon our previous studies that show that the 4T1 mouse model of TNBC develops cachexia during metastatic progression,[171] here we report the reduction of muscle mass, development of cachexia, and presence of the ZIP14-zinc axis in a novel *Bard1*-deficient orthotopic metastatic model of murine *Brca*-like TNBC.

Female individuals harboring loss of function mutations in their breast cancer susceptibility proteins 1 and 2 (BRCA1/2) and the "BRCA-like" BRCA1-associated RING domain 1 (BARD1) protein are predisposed a 65% risk of developing BC by 70 years of age and represent 20% of all hereditary/familial BC cases.[201] *BRCA*-mutations are present in about 30% of TNBC patients and about 80% of *BRCA*-mutant BCs are TNBCs.[202,203] Furthermore, *BRCA*-mutant BC patients are associated with increased tumor size, histological grade, and poorer ten-year survival rate (66%) when compared to non-*BRCA*-mutant BC patients (81%).[204] Functionally, BRCA1 and BARD1 dimerize into a heterodimer, which is a critical regulator of DNA homologous recombination and double stranded-break repair pathways.[205,206] Therefore, *BRCA*- or *BRCA*-like mutant carriers, who only carry one functional copy of the *BRCA* or *BARD1* gene, respectively, that undergo loss of heterozygosity through acquired loss of function mutations in their functional *BRCA/BARD* gene copy exhibit impaired DNA repair pathways and are more susceptible to acquisition of mutations that lead to the onset of BC.

Initial attempts to generate heterozygous or homozygous $BRCA^{null}$ GEMMs of *BRCA*-mutant BC were unsuccessful due to the lack of tumor development in the former and embryonic lethality in the latter models.[207] A breakthrough was achieved by the Baer lab, in which homozygous conditional mammary epithelium knockout *Bard1*[flex1/flex1], *Wap*[cre+] mice were generated by crossing mice with *loxP* sites flanking exon 1 of *Bard1* (*Bard1*[flex1/flex1]) with knockin mice expressing *cre* recombinase under the mammary epithelium-specific *Wap* promoter (*Wap*[cre+]).[208,209] These *Bard1*[flex1/flex1], *Wap*[cre+] mice exhibit no developmental defects and develop spontaneous mammary carcinomas with a latency of about 473 days that histologically recapitulate human *BRCA*-mutant/*BRCA*-like basal TNBC.[208,209]

3.2 Generation and validation of a *Bard1*-deficient orthotopic mouse model of *BRCA*-mutant triple-negative breast cancer cachexia

To determine the mechanisms mediating *BRCA*-like TNBC-induced cachexia, we generated a metastatic orthotopic model of *Bard1*-deficient murine TNBC by injecting 5 x 10^5 *Bard1*-deficient tumor cells, isolated from the primary mammary carcinomas of *Bard1*[flex1/flex1], *Wap*[cre+] mice, into the fourth mammary fat pad of 8- to 9- week old syngeneic female B6129SF1/J mice (Figure 3-1A). These mice developed primary mammary carcinomas that metastasized to the lungs along with concomitant reduction of body weight and loss of muscle mass and function, measured by hind-limb grip strength prior to tumor cell injection and at endpoint, compared to healthy control mice (Figure 3-1B-D). Pathological analysis of GAST muscles showed histological signs of muscle atrophy in the GAST muscles from orthotopic *Bard1*-deficient metastatic TNBC models compared to control mice (Figure 3-1E). Subsequent measurements of GAST muscle fiber CSA revealed that orthotopic *Bard1*-deficient metastatic TNBC models had a larger percentage of muscle fibers with smaller CSA and smaller percentage of muscle fibers with larger CSA compared to healthy control mice (Figure 3-1F). To further confirm the presence of muscle atrophy and cachexia, RT-qPCR revealed that GAST, DIA, TA, and heart muscles from orthotopic *Bard1*-deficient metastatic TNBC models exhibited elevated expression of *Murf1*, *Mafbx*, *Fbxo31*, and *Musa1* muscle atrophy-associated E3 ubiquitin ligases when compared to healthy control mice (Figure 3-1G). Taken together, these results suggest that orthotopic *Bard1*-deficient metastatic TNBC models develop metastatic disease along with a concomitant development of cachexia.

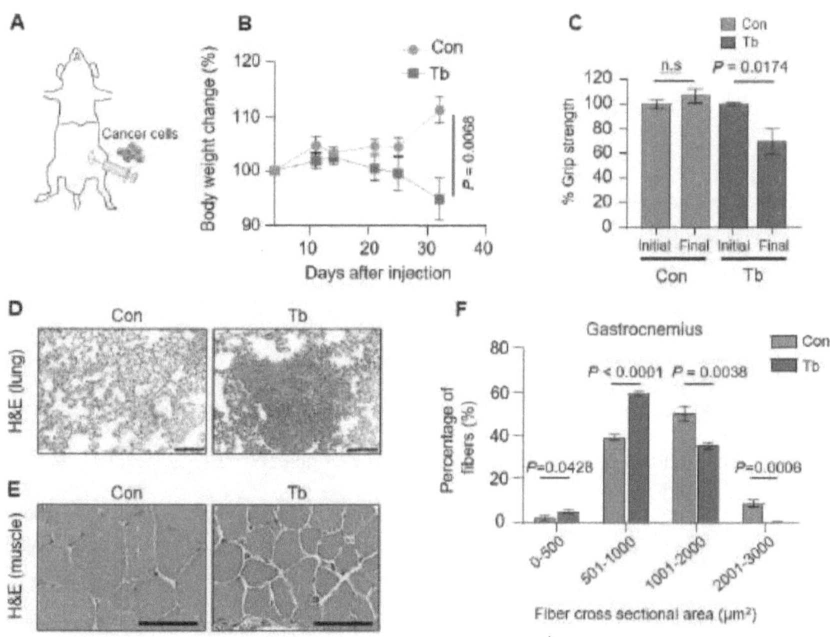

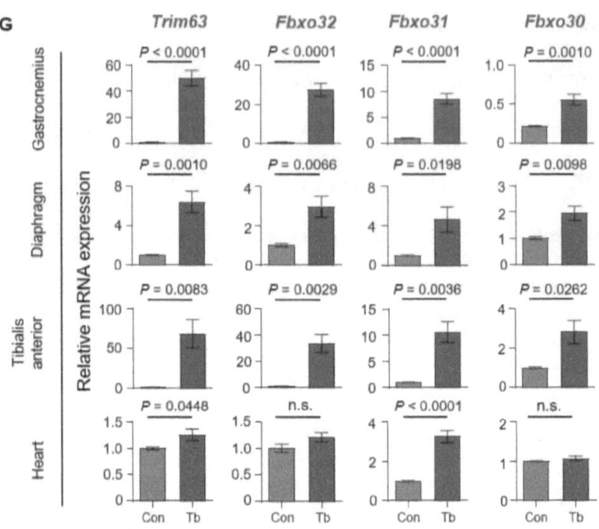

Figure 3-1: Cachexia development in a *Bard1*-deficient mouse model of *Brca*-like triple-negative breast cancer (TNBC)

(**A**) Schematic depicting the orthotopic injection of 5 x 10^5 *Bard1*-deficient TNBC cells into the left fourth mammary fat pad of 8- to 9- week old female syngeneic B6129SF1/J mice. (**B**) Measurements and analysis of body weight of healthy non tumor-bearing control (Con, grey lines) mice compared to tumor-bearing (Tb, blue lines) *Bard1*-deficient TNBC models post tumor cell injection. (**C**) Measurements of hind-limb grip strength in orthotopic *Bard1*-deficient metastatic TNBC models (Tb, blue bars) compared to control mice (Con, gray bars) before tumor-cell injection (initial) and at endpoint (final). Data is normalized to the mean of initial values of each group. (**D**) Representative images of hematoxylin and eosin- (H&E) stained lung tissue sections from orthotopic *Bard1*-deficient metastatic TNBC models compared to control mice. Scale bars represent 100 μm. (**E**) Representative images of H&E-stained gastrocnemius muscle cross-sections from *Bard1*-deficient TNBC mice compared to control mice. Scale bars represent 50 μm. (**F**) Quantitation of gastrocnemius muscle fiber cross-sectional area (CSA) from orthotopic *Bard1*-deficient metastatic TNBC models compared to control mice. Morphometric analysis is shown as the distribution frequency of muscle fibers by CSA. (**G**) Results from real-time quantitative reverse transcription PCR (RT-qPCR) analysis of muscle atrophy markers *Trim63* (*Murf1*), *Fbxo32* (*Mafbx*), *Fbxo31*, and *Fbxo30* (*Musa1*) in the gastrocnemius muscles from orthotopic *Bard1*-deficient metastatic TNBC models compared to control mice. $n = 5$ mice/group. Data are expressed as mean $\pm$ standard error of the mean (SEM). *p*-values were determined by the two-tailed, unpaired Student's *t* test. Con, control; Tb, tumor-bearing; *n.s.,* not significant.

3.3 The zinc-importer gene, *Zip14*, and zinc-inducible genes, *Mt1* and *Mt2*, are systemically upregulated in multiple cachectic muscle groups in the *Bard1*-deficient mouse model of *Brca*-like triple-negative breast cancer

Our previous studies have revealed that aberrant upregulation of *Zip14* expression in muscle cells and intramuscular zinc concentrations are associated with and mediate metastasis-induced cachexia in metastatic mouse models of PDAC, BC, colon, and lung cancer.[171,185] To determine whether development of cachexia in the orthotopic *Bard1*-deficient metastatic TNBC model is associated with upregulated *Zip14* and zinc concentration in cachectic muscles, we performed RT-qPCR in the cachectic GAST muscles *for Zip14*, and zinc-inducible *Mt1* and *Mt2* genes from orthotopic *Bard1*-deficient metastatic TNBC models and healthy control mice. In line with our previous studies, we found that *Zip14*, *Mt1*, and *Mt2* were all upregulated in the cachectic GAST muscles of orthotopic *Bard1*-deficient metastatic TNBC models and compared to control mice (Figure 3-2). To confirm the systemic presence of the aberrantly upregulated *Zip14* and *Mt* expression, we repeated the RT-qPCR on DIA, TA, and heart muscles and found that these genes were similarly upregulated in these muscle groups from orthotopic *Bard1*-deficient metastatic TNBC models and compared to control mice (Figure 3-3).

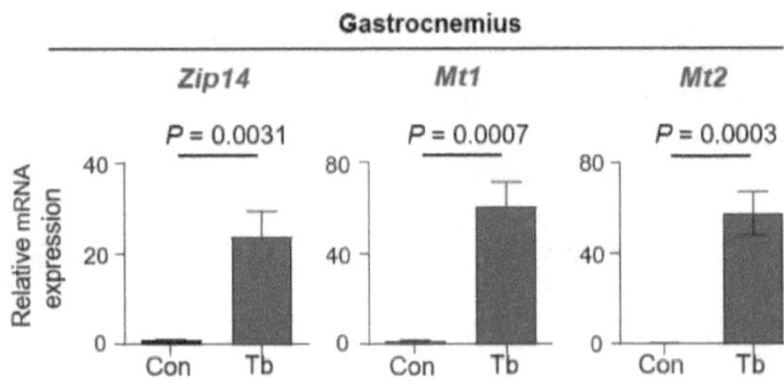

Figure 3.2: *Zip14* and zinc-inducible genes, *Mt1* and *Mt2*, expression are upregulated in the cachectic gastrocnemius muscles in the *Bard1*-deficient mouse model of *Brca*-like triple-negative breast cancer (TNBC)

Results from RT-qPCR analysis of *Zip14, Mt1*, and *Mt2,* expression in the gastrocnemius muscles from orthotopic *Bard1*-deficient metastatic TNBC models (Tb, blue bars) compared to control mice (Con, gray bars) The mouse *Gapdh* gene was utilized as an internal control. $n = 5$ mice/group. Data are expressed as mean $\pm$ standard error of the mean (SEM). *p*-values were determined by the two-tailed, unpaired Student's t-test. Con, control; Tb, tumor-bearing.

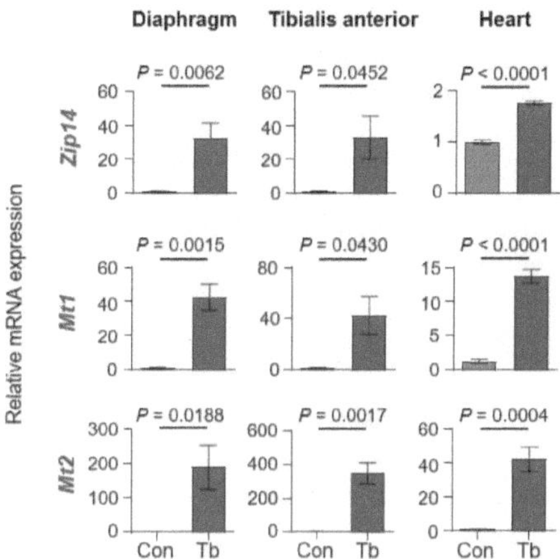

Figure 3-3: *Zip14* and zinc-inducible genes, *Mt1* and *Mt2*, expression are upregulated in diaphragm, tibialis anterior, and heart muscles in the *Bard1*-deficient mouse model of *Brca*-like triple-negative breast cancer (TNBC)

Results from RT-qPCR analysis of *Zip14, Mt1*, and *Mt2*, expression in the diaphragm, tibilalis anterior, and heart muscles from orthotopic *Bard1*-deficient metastatic TNBC models (Tb, blue bars) compared to control mice (Con, gray bars) The mouse *Gapdh* gene was utilized as an internal control. n = 5 mice/group. Data are expressed as mean ± standard error of the mean (SEM). p-values were determined by the two-tailed, unpaired Student's t-test. Con, Control; Tb, tumor-bearing.

3.4 Upregulation of Zip14 is associated with elevated zinc concentration in cachectic muscles in the *Bard1*-deficient mouse model of *Brca*-like triple-negative breast cancer

To determine if elevated muscle cell *Zip14* expression is associated with a concomitant increase of intracellular metal ion concentrations, we performed ICP-MS for Zn^{2+}, Fe^{2+}, Mn^{2+} and Cu^{2+} on muscle cell lysate taken from the GAST and DIA muscles from orthotopic *Bard1*-deficient metastatic TNBC models and healthy control mice. The results revealed that the cachectic GAST and DIA muscles from orthotopic *Bard1*-deficient metastatic TNBC models had elevated Zn^{2+} and Fe^{2+} concentrations compared to control mice (Figure 3-4). Furthermore, Mn^{2+} and Cu^{2+} concentrations were found to be increased only in GAST, but not DIA muscles. These results suggest that elevated ZIP14 expression in cachectic GAST and DIA muscles of orthotopic *Bard1*-deficient metastatic TNBC mice functions in its canonical role as a Zn^{2+} importer and possibly as a Fe^{2+} importer as well. The lack of increased Mn^{2+} and Cu^{2+} concentrations in cachectic DIA muscles suggests that these two metal ions may be imported via a different metal ion importer and may be independent of cachexia induction.

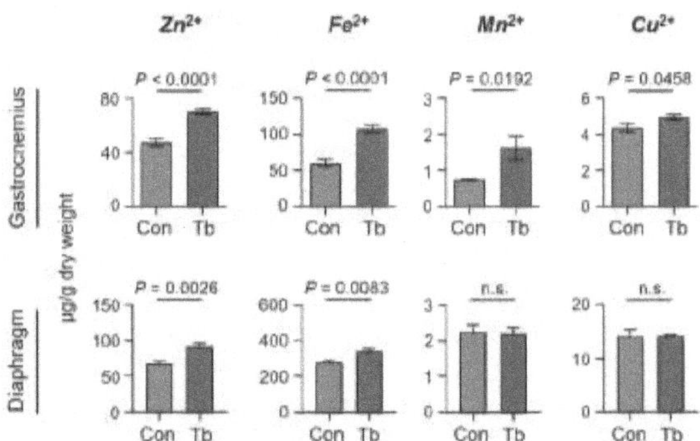

Figure 3-4: Intramuscular zinc and iron levels are elevated in the cachectic gastrocnemius and diaphragm muscles from the *Bard1*-deficient mouse model of *Brca*-like triple-negative breast cancer (TNBC)

Results from metal ion analysis by ICP-MS of zinc (Zn^{2+}), iron (Fe^{2+}), manganese (Mn^{2+}), and copper (Cu^{2+}) on gastrocnemius and diaphragm muscles from orthotopic *Bard1*-deficient metastatic TNBC models (Tb, blue bars) compared to control (Con, grey bars) mice at endpoint. Results are shown as micrograms (mg) of metal ions per gram (g) of muscle dry weight. *n = 7* mice for gastrocnemius muscles. *n = 7* Con mice and *n = 6* Tb mice for diaphragm muscles. Data are expressed as mean $\pm$ standard error of the mean (SEM). *p*-values were determined by the two-tailed, unpaired Student's t-test. Con, Control; Tb, tumor-bearing; *n.s.*, not significant.

3.5 Elevated *Zip14* expression is associated with increased SMAD2 signaling in the cachectic gastrocnemius muscles from the *Bard1*-deficient mouse model of *Brca*-like triple-negative breast cancer

Our previous studies in metastatic mouse models of BC, colon, and lung cancer revealed that tumor-associated TGF-β signaling induces muscle cell expression of *Zip14* through the activation of the NF-κB pathway via phosphorylation of downstream SMAD2 proteins.[171] To determine if the SMAD2 pathway is activated concomitant with elevated Zip14 expression in the cachectic muscles of orthotopic *Bard1*-deficient metastatic TNBC models, we performed an immunoblot analysis for phospho-SMAD2, SMAD2, and skeletal actin. Immunoblot analysis confirmed that elevated *Zip14* occurs concomitant with elevated SMAD2 phosphorylation in the cachectic GAST muscles of orthotopic *Bard1*-deficient metastatic TNBC models when compared to control mice (Figure 3-5). Taken together, this suggests that TGF-β mediated SMAD2 phosphorylation is associated with elevated *Zip14* expression and increased intramuscular zinc concentration in the cachectic muscles of orthotopic *Bard1*-deficient metastatic TNBC models.

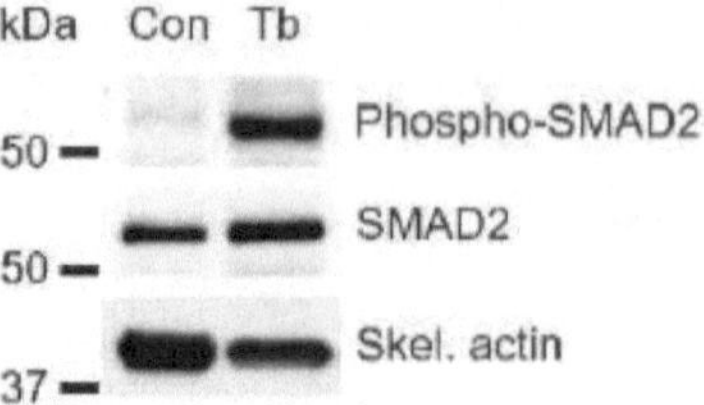

Figure 3-5: Protein levels of phospho-SMAD2 are elevated in the cachectic gastrocnemius muscles from the *Bard1*-deficient mouse model of *Brca*-like triple-negative breast cancer (TNBC)

Immunoblot analysis probing for phospho-SMAD2, SMAD2, and skeletal actin (Skel. actin) in gastrocnemius muscle-cell lysate from orthotopic *Bard1*-deficient metastatic TNBC models (Tb, right) compared to control (Con, left) mice. Skel. actin was used as an internal control. Data is representative of three independent experiments. Con, Control; Tb, tumor-bearing.

3.6 Discussion

Continuing our studies that show that an aberrant *Zip14*/zinc axis is associated with metastatic PDAC, BC, colon, and lung cancer-induced cachexia;[171,185] here, we report and characterize the development of cachexia a novel orthotopic metastasis mouse model of *Brca*-like TNBC that similarly develops cachexia along with concomitant presence of a *Zip14*/zinc axis in cachectic muscles. The orthotopic implantation of *Bard1*-deficient TNBC cells into the mammary glands of syngeneic mice resulted in the growth of mammary tumors that histologically recapitulate human *BRCA*-mutant TNBC and spontaneously metastasizes to the lungs along with the progressive development of muscle atrophy and cachexia. Although it remains to be determined if *BRCA*-mutant BC patients exhibit elevated risk of cachexia, the orthotopic *Bard1*-deficient metastatic TNBC mouse model represents a useful preclinical model to elucidate the mechanisms mediating metastasis and cachexia development in *BRCA*-mutant TNBC. Furthermore, CT-imaging can be utilized to determine the prevalence of cachexia in *BRCA*-mutant BC patients.

In addition to studies on cachexia, the orthotopic *Bard1*-deficient metastatic TNBC mouse model also represents a useful preclinical model to study the mechanisms of poly (ADP-ribose) polymerase (PARP) inhibitors in *BRCA*-mutant BC.[210] Because *BRCA*-mutant BCs have impaired DNA homologous recombination and double stranded-break repair mechanisms and PARP functions in DNA damage sensing and single-stand DNA repair, PARP inhibitors in *BRCA*-mutant BCs cripple the tumor cell's ability to efficiently execute high fidelity DNA repair, leading to accumulation of DNA damage and cell death.[202] PARP inhibitors are currently approved for treatment of *BRCA1/2*-mutant BCs. Furthermore, there are ongoing clinical trials elucidating the efficacy of PARP inhibitors on patients with sporadic TNBC with "BRCA-like" similarities to *BRCA*-mutant BCs, and the *Bard1*-mutant mouse model can help facilitate the testing of PARP inhibitor efficacy in TNBC patients with *BRCA*-like mutations.[211,212] In addition, it was been reported that PARP activation in the muscles of mouse models of lung cancer-induced cachexia may promote cachexia as deletion of PARP1/2 results in the rescue of body weight loss and reduces muscle expression of muscle proteolysis genes.[213] Future studies are needed to elucidate the effects of PARP inhibitors on *BRCA*-like BC-associated cachexia.

Here, we report that the systemic upregulation of *Zip14* expression in multiple muscle groups and concomitant increase in intramuscular zinc are associated with the development of cachexia in the orthotopic *Bard1*-deficient metastatic mouse model. Unexpectedly, we also found that intramuscular iron levels were also increased along with marginal increases of manganese and copper, which were not found in our previous studies associating the *Zip14*/zinc axis in mouse models of PDAC, BC, colon, and lung cancer. Regardless, taken together, our study findings suggest that treatment with ZIP14 inhibitors and metal chelation therapy to lower intramuscular zinc and other metal ions should be tested in preclinical cancer-induced cachexia models. Future studies are warranted to evaluate if these strategies can reduce cachexia, rescue muscle mass and function, and extend survival in the orthotopic *Bard1*-deficient metastatic mouse model.

In addition to targeting *Zip14* expression and intramuscular zinc, it is also essential to identify factors that induce *Zip14* expression in the cachectic muscles of the orthotopic *Bard1*-deficient metastatic TNBC mouse model. We had previously shown *in vitro* that tumor-associated TGF-β induces *Zip14* expression in muscle cells and myoblasts through phosphorylation of SMAD2 and that *in vivo* treatment of cachectic mouse models of BC and colon cancer with a TGF-β inhibitor reduced muscle atrophy and intramuscular SMAD2 phosphorylation and *Zip14* expression.[185] Here, we report similar elevated SMAD2 phosphorylation in the cachectic muscles of the orthotopic *Bard1*-deficient metastatic TNBC mouse model. Although our findings do not confirm that a TGF-β/phospho-SMAD2 mechanism induces *Zip14* expression cachexia, TGF-β inhibitors should be tested in the orthotopic *Bard1*-deficient metastatic TNBC mouse model to evaluate if the treatment could reduce SMAD2 phosphorylation, *Zip14* expression, and muscle atrophy. Taken together, future studies are needed to determine targetable factors that induce intramuscular *Zip14* expression and to test the efficacy of ZIP14 inhibitors and metal ion chelation strategies to reduce muscle atrophy and cachexia in the orthotopic *Bard1*-deficient metastatic TNBC mouse model.

Chapter 4: Tumor-infiltrating B cells promote the invasion of lung metastases in triple-negative breast cancer mouse models though upregulation of p-mTOR

Triple-negative breast cancer and metastasis

In the USA, BC is the most frequently diagnosed cancer and it is estimated that 284,200 new cases will be diagnosed along with 44,130 deaths in 2021.[2,173] Although 6% of BC patients are diagnosed with stage IV metastatic disease due to routine early screening protocols, it is estimated that 30% of patients diagnosed with early-stage BC eventually develop distant metastases, even years after successful mastectomy or treatment of the primary tumor.[214,215] BC is well documented as a heterogenous disease that is characterized into four major subtypes based on estrogen receptor (ER), progesterone receptor (PR), or human epidermal growth factor 2 (HER2) expression: luminal A (ER^+ and/or PR^+, $HER2^-$), luminal B (ER^+ and/or PR^+, $HER2^{+/-}$), HER2-enriched (ER^-, PR^-, $HER2^+$), and TNBC (ER^-, PR^-, $HER2^-$).[215]

In particular, TNBC, which accounts for about 20% of all BC cases, presents with higher tumor grade, lymph node positivity, mitotic count, and greater metastatic potential, which all culminates in poorer prognosis and increased mortality compared to other subtypes (TNBC: 42%; other subtypes: 28%).[216-218] Furthermore, TNBC is associated with elevated risk of visceral metastases (lung and brain), which have higher mortality rates compared to bone metastases.[217-219] Lung and brain metastases comprise 32% and 9% of total TNBC metastases compared to a range of 21-25.5% and 4-8% in non-TNBC subtypes, respectively.[219] Because TNBCs lacks overexpression of ER, PR, and HER2, treatments used in other BC subtypes that target these receptors cannot be used to treat TNBC patients. While chemotherapy remains a mainstay of TNBC treatments, TNBC exhibits higher chemoresistance compared to other BC subtypes, resulting in a mOS of 13.3 months.[220] Furthermore, clinical studies report that about 50% of early-stage or localized TNBC patients treated successfully with mastectomy exhibit significant RCB

(RCB-II or RCB-III), which correspond with 55% and 23% 10-year relapse-free survival rates, respectively.[221,222] Likewise, TNBC patients also have elevated distant recurrence rates (6.7-10.5%) compared to overall BC patients (2.1-6.4%).[223] Taken together, TNBC exhibit an elevated risk of developing metastatic disease compared to other BC subtypes, which underscores the importance of elucidating the various mechanisms promoting TNBC metastasis to identify potential targets for the treatment of or prevention of mTNBC.

Spatial localization of non-tumor cells in the tumor microenvironment is associated with anti- or pro-tumor function

The TME is a complex and heterogenous microenvironment comprised of a multitude of non-tumor stromal and immune cells, including myeloid and lymphocyte populations. Simply evaluating the average densities of immune cell infiltrates in tumor tissues may overlook the significance of spatial heterogeneity and mask the effects of spatial distribution of specific immune populations.[224] Moreover, many clinical studies utilize tissue microarrays, which only represent a small area of a tumor and may not be representative of the entire tumor overall.[93] However, there is growing interest in the field of immune cell topography and spatial localization in the TME and studies have shown that the density and spatial localization of stromal or immune cells as intratumoral, stromal, or at the invasive margin, in BC can be utilized as biomarkers with positive or negative prognostic value.[225-228] Pollard et al, revealed that that tumor-associated macrophages localized at the invasive margin can enhance the motility of lung metastasis by secreting epidermal growth factor (EGF) in the PyMT GEMM of BC.[225,226] Another study in BC patients revealed that high stromal macrophage density was associated with larger tumor size and higher mitotic count when compared to intratumoral macrophages; while intratumoral macrophages, and not stromal macrophages, were directly and significantly correlated with microvessel density.[229] In addition, Gao et al, demonstrated that fibroblasts isolated specifically from the invasive margin of human BC patients significantly increased EMT and motility of human luminal and TNBC cell lines when compared to fibroblasts isolated from intratumoral or distal normal tissue zones.[227]

Spatial localization of CD8$^+$ TILs have also been shown to influence clinical outcome. In BC patients, high TIL density at the invasive margin is associated with smaller tumor sizes post chemotherapy and high intratumoral TILs are associated with improved prognosis and mOS.[230,231] Conversely, breast tumors with TILs absent from the stromal and intratumoral locations and restricted only to the invasive margin or peritumoral areas are associated with a more immunosuppressive and fibrotic TME and poor prognosis.[230] Furthermore, breast tumors with TILs absent from the intratumoral region and restricted only to stromal compartments are associated with high infiltration of pro-tumorigenic neutrophils, an immunosuppressive TME, and worse prognosis.[230]

A recent study analyzed the association between TIBs in TNBC primary tumors and RFS revealed that the density of CD20$^+$ B cells in the stroma between tumor cell nests does not significantly correlate with RFS.[93] The study also revealed that increased abundance of spatially dispersed TIBs and LC-Bs within the tumor nests of TNBC primary tumors were associated with improved RFS, suggesting that TIBs within tumor nests are functionally distinct from TIBs in the stroma between tumor cell nests. Taken together, these findings reveal that the spatial localization of non-tumor cells in the TME can exhibit differing and unique functions associated with their particular region. Although there is growing interest in elucidating the link between spatial localization, function, and effects on patient prognosis of non-tumor cells in primary tumors, there remains a lack of similar studies focusing on the metastatic context.

4.2 B220[+] B cells are recruited to the invasive margin of lung metastases in mouse models and patients with triple-negative breast cancer

To determine the spatial localization of various immune cell populations in TNBC lung metastases, we generated allograft orthotopic and experimental metastasis models of TNBC using the murine TNBC cells lines: 4T1 and LM3. The two cells lines were specifically selected based off of three criteria: 1) a highly aggressive basal TNBC subtype with 2) the ability to accurately model, recapitulate, and spontaneously metastasize to the same sites (with the highest metastatic potential to the lung) as human TNBC patients when implanted into an immunocompetent host, and 3) distinct mutational landscapes between the cell lines to eliminate mutation- or cell line-specific phenotypes.[232-234] To generate 4T1 and LM3 orthotopic and experimental metastasis models, we injected 5×10^5 4T1 or 1×10^6 LM3 cells into the left mammary fat pad or 1×10^5 4T1 or LM3 cells into the tail vein of 6- to 8-week old female syngeneic BALB/cJ mice, respectively (Figure 4-1A, B). Both 4T1 and LM3 orthotopic metastasis models developed primary TNBCs that spontaneously metastasized to the lungs and the experimental metastasis models developed lung metastases in the absence of a primary tumor (Figure 4-1A, B).

A
Orthotopic metastasis model
Tumor growth
And lung metastasis
Tumor cells
B
Experimental metastasis model
Lung metastasi
Tumor cells
C
4T1 experimental metastasis model
B220
S100A9
D
4T1 orthotopic metastasis model
4T1 experimental metastasis model
B220
CD3
IBA1
DAPI
Merged
E
Orthotopic metastasis model
4T1
LM3
B220
F
Invasive margin
Interior
B220+ cell density (% total)
100
75
50
25
0
4T1
LM3
G
Experimental metastasis model
4T1
LM3
B220
H
B220+ cell density (% total)
100
75
50
25
0
4T1
LM3
I
Human lung metastasis
High TIB
Low TIB
CD20
J
CD20+ cell density (% total)
100
75
50
25
0
Edge Interior

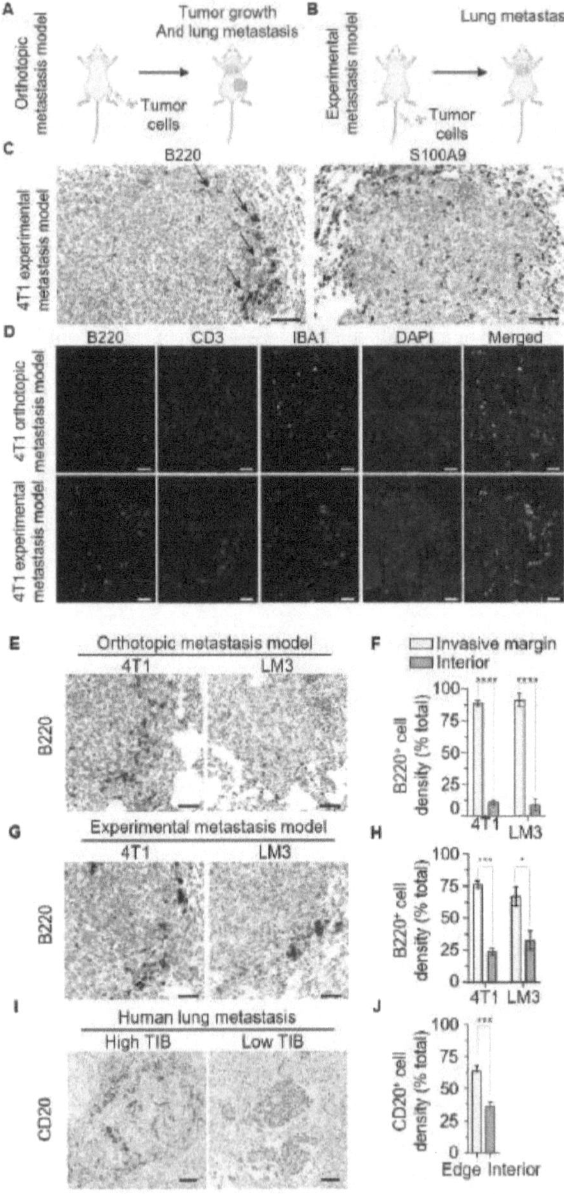

72

Figure 4-1: B cells localize at the invasive margin of lung metastases in triple-negative breast cancer models and patients.

(**A**) 4T1 and LM3 orthotopic metastasis models were generated by orthotopic injection of 5×10^5 4T1 and 1×10^6 LM3 cells into the left fourth mammary fat pad of 6- to 8-week old female syngeneic BALB/cJ background mice. 4T1 and LM3 orthotopic metastasis models developed mammary tumors that spontaneously metastasized to the lungs. (**B**) 4T1 and LM3 experimental metastasis models were generated by intravenous injection of 1×10^5 4T1 or LM3 cells into the tail vein of 6- to 8-week old female syngeneic BALB/cJ background mice. 4T1 and LM3 experimental metastasis models developed lung metastases. (**C**) Representative images of metastatic lung sections from 4T1 experimental metastasis models immunostained using antibodies against B220 for B cells (left) and S100A9 for neutrophils (right). Black arrows mark representative B220$^+$ B cells located at the invasive margin of lung metastasis. Scale bar represents 50μm. (**D**) Representative images of metastatic lung sections from 4T1 orthotopic metastasis (top) and experimental (bottom) metastasis models immunostained using antibodies against B220 for B cells (green), CD3 for T cells (red), and IBA1 for macrophages (far red). Scale Bars represent 100μm. (**E-H**) Representative images of metastatic lung sections from 4T1 and LM3 orthotopic (**E**) and experimental (**G**) metastasis models immunostained using antibodies against B220 for B cells. Scale bars represents 50μm. Bar graphs represent metastasis-infiltrating B cells by localization, either at the invasive margin or interior of lung metastases, and calculated as a proportion of total metastasis-infiltrating B cells in 4T1 and LM3 orthotopic (**F**) and experimental (**H**) metastasis model lungs. n = 7 mice for 4T1 orthotopic metastasis models. n = 4 mice for LM3 orthotopic metastasis models. n = 3 mice for 4T1 and LM3 experimental metastasis models. (**I, J**) Representative images of metastatic lung sections from human TNBC patients with confirmed lung metastases and immunostained using antibodies against CD20 and shown as high (left) and low (right) density. Scale bars represent 100μm. Bars graphs representing tumor-infiltrating CD20$^+$ B cells (TIBs) by localization, either at the invasive margin or interior of lung metastases, and calculated as a proportion of total CD20$^+$ TIBs.

n = 7 human TNBC patients. In all panels, data is expressed as mean ± the standard error of the mean. p-values were determined by the two-tailed, unpaired Student's t-test. TIB, tumor-infiltrating B cell. * $p<0.05$, ** $p<0.01$, *** $p<0.001$, **** $p<0.0001$

To determine the spatial localization of metastasis-infiltrating immune cell populations, we first stained metastatic lungs from 4T1 experimental metastasis models for B220$^+$ B cells and S100A9$^+$ neutrophils (Figure 4-1C). Our results revealed an interesting discrepancy in the pattern and localization between B220$^+$ B cells and S100A9$^+$ neutrophils. The metastasis-infiltrating neutrophils were found to be evenly distributed throughout the metastases, but the localization of metastasis-infiltrating B cells appeared to be mostly restricted to the invasive margin of lung metastases (Figure 4-1C). To identify the spatial localization patterns of other metastasis-infiltrating immune cells, we performed multiplex immunofluorescence staining for B220$^+$ B cells, CD3$^+$ T cells, and Iba1$^+$ macrophages on metastatic lungs from both 4T1 orthotopic and experimental metastasis models (Figure 4-1D). Interestingly, we observed that metastasis-infiltrating B220$^+$ B cells remained localized to the invasive margin of lung metastases in both orthotopic and experimental metastasis models, while T cells and macrophages were eventually distributed throughout the lung metastases similarly to neutrophils. Further immunohistochemical staining for B220$^+$ B cells in the metastatic lungs of 4T1 and LM3 orthotopic metastasis and subsequent quantitative analysis of B cell spatial localization as either interior or invasive margin confirmed that 88.9-91.1% of all metastasis-infiltrating B220$^+$ B cells were localized at the invasive margin of TNBC lung metastases (Figure 4-1E, F). The quantitative analysis further revealed that the metastasis-infiltrating B cells were distributed as single TIBs and not aggregated or organized into TLSs.

It is well documented that primary tumors can modulate the stromal or immune microenvironment of distant organs to establish "premetastatic niches" that can promote metastatic colonization through the release of soluble factors and exosomes.[235] To determine whether the recruitment of localization of B220$^+$ B cells to the invasive margin of TNBC lung metastases is mediated by the presence of a primary tumor, we repeated our B220$^+$ immunohistochemistry staining on 4T1 and LM3 experimental metastasis models (Figure 4-1G). Quantitative analysis of spatial localization further confirmed that 67.2-76.3% of metastasis-infiltrating B220$^+$ B cells were localized at the invasive margin of TNBC lung metastases (Figure 4-1H). Although the proportion of B cells at the invasive margin is lower in experimental metastasis models compared to orthotopic metastasis models, the trend of preferential invasive margin localization remains unaltered. This suggests that lung metastases are inherently capable of mediating the invasive margin localization of recruited metastasis-infiltrating B cells independently of a primary tumor.

It is important to translate findings from preclinical mouse models into human patients to clinically validate that the murine phenotype accurately recapitulates that of the human disease. To this end, we analyzed the spatial localization of metastasis-infiltrating CD20$^+$ B cells in CD20-immunostained metastatic lung sections from human TNBC patients (Figure 4-1I). Spatial localization analysis revealed that 64.1% of metastasis-infiltrating CD20$^+$ B cells were localized at the invasive margin of human TNBC patient lung metastases (Figure 4-1J). Taken together, these findings suggests that B cells recruited to lung metastases are preferentially localized at the invasive margin in multiple mouse models of TNBC and human mTNBC patients.

4.3 Confirmation of metastasis-infiltrating B220[+] B cell identity

Although B220 is generally regarded as a murine pan-B cell marker, there is evidence that shows it can be aberrantly expressed on populations of plasmacytoid dendritic cells (pDCs) in mouse models of BC and human BC patients.[236,237] To confirm whether metastasis-infiltrating B220[+] B cells are bona-fide B cells or aberrant B220[+] pDCs, we performed an immunofluorescence co-stain for B220 and PAX-5 on metastatic lung sections from 4T1 and LM3 orthotopic and experimental metastasis models (Figure 2A, C). PAX-5 is a transcriptional factor that functions on as a master regulator of commitment to B cell lineage, development, and maintenance of B cell identity.[238] Although PAX-5 expression, along with B220 and CD20, is repressed upon B cell differentiation into antibody-secreting PCs, PAX-5 is exclusively expressed in and is determinative of B cell identity.[238] Quantitative analysis of metastasis-infiltrating B220[+] B cells as either PAX-5[+] or PAX5[-] confirmed that about 80-92% of B220[+] B cells are bona-fide PAX-5[+] B cells over all 4T1 and LM3 orthotopic and experimental metastasis models (Figure 2B, D). These data validates that the majority of metastasis-infiltrating B220[+] B cells are predominantly PAX-5[+] bona-fide B cells and not pDCs or other cell populations that aberrantly express B220.

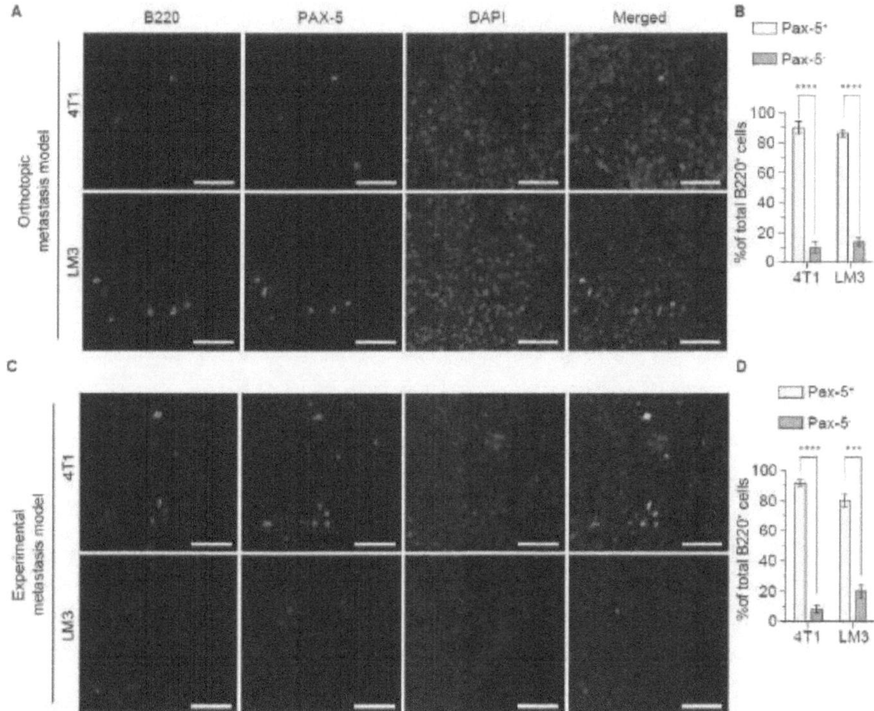

Figure 4.2: Confirmation of the identity of metastasis-infiltrating B cells by PAX-5 and B220 dual staining

(**A-D**) Representative images of lung sections from 4T1 and LM3 orthotopic (**A**) and experimental (**C**) metastasis models immunostained using antibodies against B220 (green) and PAX-5 (red). Cell nuclei are stained with DAPI. Scale bars represent 30µm. Bar graphs represent the quantitation and scoring of B220⁺ metastasis-infiltrating B cells, either as PAX-5⁺ or PAX-5⁻, as a proportion of total metastasis-infiltrating B cells in the lungs of 4T1 and LM3 orthoptic (**B**) and experimental (**D**) metastasis models. $n = 4$ mice for 4T1 and LM3 orthotopic models. $n = 3$ mice for 4T1 and

LM3 experimental metastasis models. In all panels, data is expressed as mean ± the standard error of the mean. p-values were determined by the two-tailed, unpaired Student's t-test. **** $p<0.0001$

4.4 B220[+] B cells isolated from the lungs or peripheral blood of triple-negative breast cancer mouse models promote the invasion of lung metastasis-derived organoids

Previous studies have suggested that spatial localization in the TME can affect cell function and that TIBs distributed as single cells and not in a TLS are associated with pro-tumor functions.[90,225-227] This suggests that the single cell metastasis-infiltrating B220[+] B cells localized at the invasive margin of TNBC lung metastases may exhibit tumor-promoting functions. Localization at the invasive margin is significant because it contains a distinct population of motile and migrating tumor cells that actively invade into the host tissue.[239]

To determine whether metastasis-infiltrating B cells can directly affect tumor cells, we designed a 3-dimensional (3D) organotypic co-culture invasion assay using 4T1 and LM3 lung metastasis-derived organoids and B220[+] B cells isolated from the metastatic lungs of 4T1 and LM3 orthotopic metastasis mouse models. 4T1 and LM3 lung metastasis-derived organoids were generated by subjecting respective lungs with macroscopic metastatic nodules to limited mechanical and enzymatic dissociation into microscopic cell clusters, which are then embedded into a matrigel matrix and passaged until only lung metastasis-tumor organoids remained (Figure 4-3A). The advantage of using lung metastasis-derived organoids is that they better recapitulate the 3D *in vivo* pathophysiological growth and invasion of lung metastases and their interactions with the microenvironment compared to traditional 2D cell cultures.[240] Furthermore, because these organoids were derived from lung metastases, they have undergone "metastatic selection" and have acquired intrinsic metastasis-specific alterations that are not present in their parental cell lines.[15,16] These 4T1 and LM3 lung metastasis-derived organoids were co-cultured with $1x10^4$ B220[+] B cells isolated from the metastatic lungs of respective 4T1 and LM3 orthotopic metastasis models (Figure 4-3B, C). Both monoculture control and co-cultured organoids were imaged at 0, 48, and 96 hours post embedding and the fold change in each organoid's form factor over time was calculated as a measurement of invasion into the Matrigel matrix.[241]

The results revealed a striking phenotype, in which the 4T1 and LM3 lung metastasis-derived organoids co-cultured with respective metastatic lung-isolated B220[+] B cells displayed a significant increase in form factor fold change and invasion from 48 to 96 hours post embedding compared to monocultured control organoids (Figures 4-3B, C, F, G). Visually, co-cultured lung-metastasis-derived organoids displayed increased elliptical architecture along with longer and more invasive protrusions (Figures 4-3B, C). Interestingly 4T1 and LM3 lung metastasis-derived organoids co-cultured with B220[+] B cells isolated from the peripheral blood of 4T1 and LM3 orthotopic metastasis models also exhibited an increase in form factor and invasion from 48 to 96 hours post-embedding compared to monocultured organoids (Figure 4-3D, E, H, I). These data suggest that peripheral B cells that are recruited into the TME of lung metastases can be educated and programmed by tumor cells into a tumor invasion-promoting phenotype. Moreover, because our co-cultured system only contained lung metastasis tumor cells and isolated B cells, the results suggest that this tumor invasion-promoting mechanism does not require other intermediate cells types or signaling found in the TME, and that tumor-educated B cells can independently and directly promote tumor cell invasion.

A
4T1 orthotopic metastasis model
Lung with metastasis
Dissociation
Tumor alone
Isolate B cells
Tumor + B cells
Quantify invasion of organoids

B
48 hrs
96 hrs
Org. alone
Org. + 4T1 Lung-B cells

C
48 hrs
96 hrs
Org. alone
Org. + LM3 Lung-B cells

D
48 hrs
96 hrs
Org. alone
Org. + 4T1 Blood-B cells

E
48 hrs
96 hrs
Org. alone
Org. + LM3 Blood-B cells

F
Fold change (form factor)
**
Org. alone
Org. + 4T1 lung-B cells

G
Fold change (form factor)
***
Org. alone
Org. + LM3 lung-B cells

H
Fold change (form factor)
**
Org. alone
Org. + 4T1 blood-B cells

I
Fold change (form factor)
*
Org. alone
Org. + LM3 blood-B cells

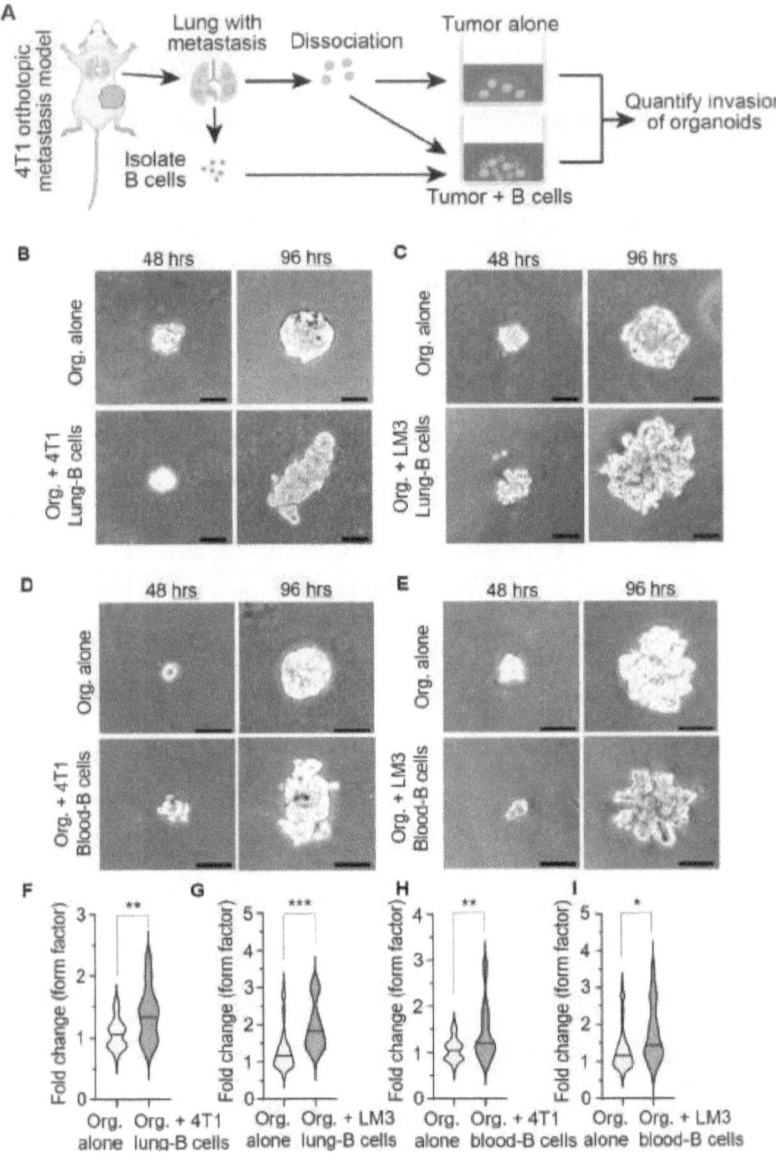

80

Figure 4-3: Lung and blood B220⁺ B cells from TNBC tumor-bearing mice enhance the invasion of lung metastasis-derived organoids

(**A**) Schematic depicting the generation of lung metastasis-derived organoids, the co-culture process, and the 3D invasion assay workflow. Lung metastasis-derived organoids were generated by harvesting lungs with macroscopic metastatic lesions from 4T1 and LM3 orthotopic metastasis models and subjecting them to mechanical and enzymatic dissociation before embedding into a Matrigel matrix. B220⁺ B cells were isolated from the metastatic lungs of 4T1 and LM3 orthotopic metastasis models using flow cytometry and added into the Matrigel matrix for co-culture with lung metastasis-derived organoids. Organoids were imaged at 0, 48, and 96 hours. (**B-E**) Representative images taken at 48 (left) and 96 (right) hours post-plating of 4T1 (**B, D**) and LM3 (**C, E**) lung metastasis-derived organoids as organoids alone (top) or co-cultured (bottom) with B220⁺ B cells isolated from the lungs (**B, C**) or peripheral blood (**D, E**) of 4T1 (**B, D**) or LM3 (**C, E**) orthotopic metastasis models. Scale bars represent 50μm. (**F-I**) Violin plots depicting the invasion of 4T1 (**F, H**) and LM3 (**G, I**) lung metastasis-derived organoids as organoids alone and co-cultured with B220+ B cells isolated from the lungs (**F, G**) or peripheral blood (**H, I**) of 4T1 (**F, H**) and LM3 (**G, I**) orthotopic metastasis models. Invasion is calculated as a measure of fold change of organoid form factor from 48 to 96 hours. n = a minimum of 9 wells for 4T1 organoid alone controls. n = 3 mice for 4T1 orthotopic metastasis model lung-isolated B220⁺ B cells. n = 1 mouse for LM3 orthotopic model lung-isolated B cells. n = 3 mice for 4T1 and LM3 orthotopic metastasis models blood-isolated B220⁺ B cells. n = 2-3 wells were plated for each co-culture of organoids and isolated B220⁺ B cells. Data is shown as the median with the violin depicting all values and p-values were determined by the unpaired Mann-Whitney U test. * $p<0.05$, ** $p<0.01$, *** $p<0.001$

4.5 B220[+] B cells isolated from the lungs of triple-negative breast cancer mouse models promotes the migration of TNBC cell lines

In addition to invasion, invasive leader tumor cells at invading fronts also undergo collective migration through the ECM and host tissue.[242] To determine whether B220[+] B cells can promote tumor cell migration, we performed a transwell migration assay using the 4T1 cell line to compare the migratory ability of tumor cells co-cultured with B220+ B cells to tumor cells alone. Tumor cells were serum-starved in serum-low media overnight and co-cultured tumor cells were co-cultured with 5×10^4 B220[+] B cells, isolated from 4T1 orthotopic metastasis models, suspended in a 0.4μm membrane transwell insert that restricts cell crossing, but not the exchange of soluble secreted factors. Transwell inserts were removed and Celltracker green-labeled tumor cells were resuspended in serum-low media in 3μm membrane transwell inserts and placed into wells containing growth medium to facilitate tumor cell migration to the basal side of the membrane (Figure 3D). Imaging and quantitative analysis of total fully migrated tumor cells on the basal membrane showed that significantly more tumor cells co-cultured with B220[+] B cells had fully migrated to through the limited-permeability membrane compared to non co-cultured tumor cells (Figure 3E, F). These data further show that B220[+] B cells isolated from TNBC tumor-bearing mice not only promote the invasion, but also migration of tumor cells *in vitro*. Interestingly, the assay results suggests that the signaling mechanism mediating the invasion and migration of tumor cells relies on secreted factors, due to the transwell insert keeping the tumor cells and B cells physically apart during the co-culture process. Further studies are needed to identify the tumor and B cell secreted factors that mediate this mechanism.

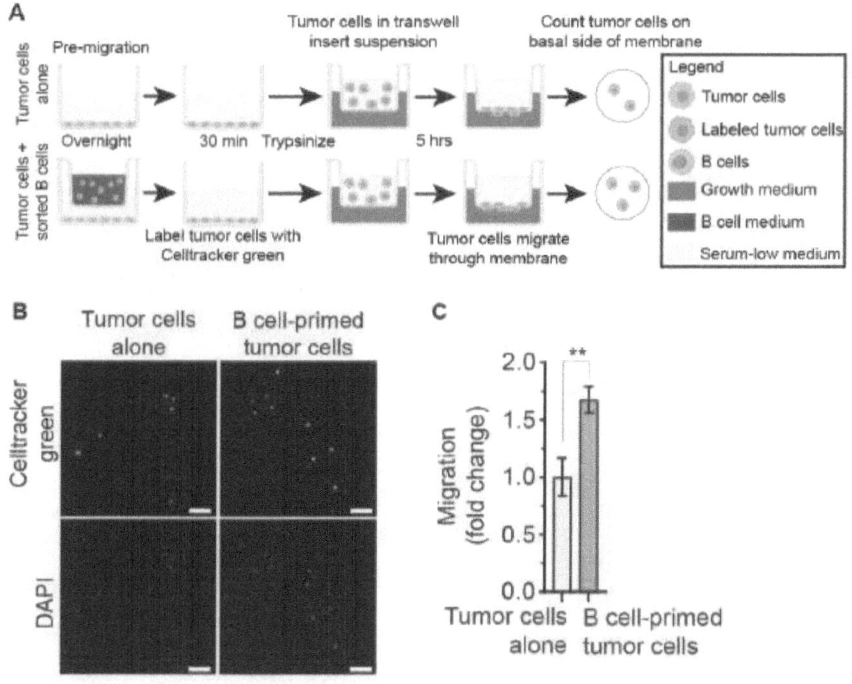

Figure 4-4: Lung B220[+] B cells isolated triple-negative breast cancer mouse models promotes the migration of TNBC cell lines

(A) Schematic of transwell migration assay workflow. 4T1 tumor cells were serum-starved overnight in serum-low media without (top) or with (bottom) B220[+] B cells sorted from the lungs of 4T1 orthotopic metastasis models in a transwell insert with a semi-permeable 0.4μm membrane containing B cell media. Inserts were removed and tumor cells were labeled with Celltracker Green at 5μM for 30min, trypsinized, and resuspended in a transwell insert containing serum-low medium with a 3μm limited-permeability membrane. Transwells were placed into wells containing growth medium and incubated for 5 hours to allow tumor cells migrate through the limited permeability membrane. Membrane were fixed paraformaldehyde, cells on the apical side were scraped off, and the membrane were excised and mounted with DAPI-containing mounting medium onto slides with basal-side up. Total migrated tumor cells on the basal side were imaged and counted for each transwell membrane. (**B**) Representative images of a 10x magnification field of view of fully migrated 4T1 tumor cells on the basal side of the membrane from 4T1 cells alone (left) and co-cultured (right) with B220$^+$ B cells isolated from the lungs of 4T1 orthotopic metastasis models. Images are representative of total fully migrated 4T1 tumor cell counts on each membrane. Scale bars represent 50μm. (**C**) Bar graphs representing the total number of fully migrated 4T1 tumor cells on the basal side of the membrane from 4T1 cells alone and co-cultured with B220$^+$ B cells isolated from the lungs of 4T1 orthotopic metastasis models. $n = 4$ tumor cell-alone controls. $n = 3$ mice for 4T1 orthotopic metastasis model lung-isolated B220$^+$ B cells. $n = 1$-3 wells per mouse for co-cultured 4T1 cells. Data is expressed as mean $\pm$ the standard error of the mean and p-values were determined by the two-tailed, unpaired Student's t-test. ** $p<0.01$

4.6 B cell-deficient mice show reduced invasive fronts and micrometastases during early metastatic disease

We further analyzed B220-stained lung sections from the 4T1 orthotopic metastasis model for association between the 1) the density of metastasis-infiltrating B cells per surface area of each metastasis and 2) number of tumor cells per metastasis and the respective proportion of metastasis-infiltrating B cells. Quantitative histological analysis revealed that micrometastases (1-50 tumor cells) and medium-metastases (51-100 tumor cells) contained increased proportions of B cells to tumor cells when compared to macrometastases (>100 tumor cells) (Figures 4-5A-C).

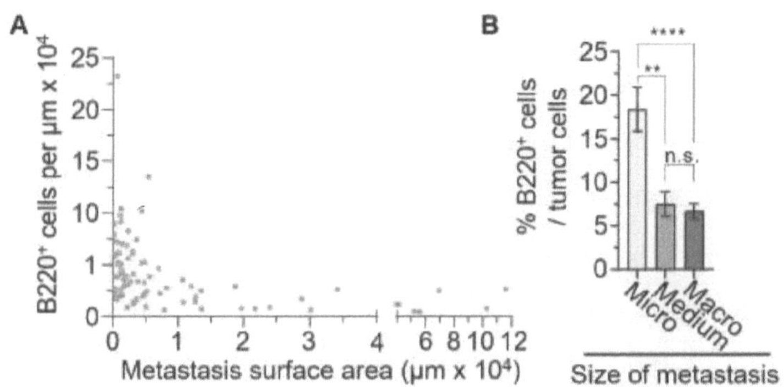
A
B220⁺ cells per µm x 10⁴
25
20
15
10
1
0
0 1 2 3 4 6 8 10 12
Metastasis surface area (µm x 10⁴)
B
****
**
n.s.
% B220⁺ cells / tumor cells
25
20
15
10
5
0
Micro
Medium
Macro
Size of metastasis

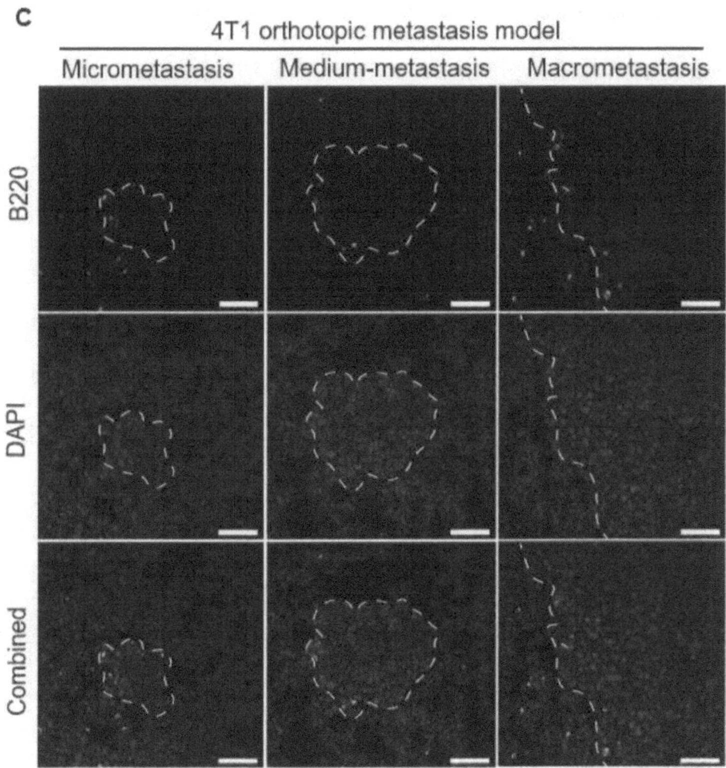
C
4T1 orthotopic metastasis model
Micrometastasis
Medium-metastasis
Macrometastasis
B220
DAPI
Combined

Figure 4-5: B cell density is elevated in smaller metastases compared to larger metastases

(**A**) Dot plot depicting the density of lung metastasis-infiltrating B220$^+$ B cells per metastasis surface area to the surface area of matching metastases. (**B**) Bar graphs depicting metastasis-infiltrating B cells as a proportion of total tumor cells from micro- (1-50 tumor cells), medium- (51-100 tumor cells), and macrometastases (>100 tumor cells) from 4T1 orthotopic metastasis models. (**C**) Representative images of lung sections containing micro (left), medium (center), and macrometastases (right) from 4T1 orthotopic metastasis models taken at 3 weeks post tumor cell injection and immunostained using antibodies against B220 (green). Cell nuclei are stained with DAPI (blue). The edge of lung metastases are outlined by the dotted white line. Scale bars represent 50μm. n = 6 for B 4T1 orthotopic metastasis models. p-values were determined by the two-tailed, unpaired Student's t-test. $n.s.$ not significant, ** $p<0.01$, **** $p<0.0001$

To evaluate the effects of metastasis-infiltrating B cells on early lung metastasis development and to validate our *in vitro* findings *in vivo*, we generated 4T1 orthotopic metastasis models using syngeneic immunocompetent B cell-proficient (B-proficient) BALB/cJ and B cell-deficient Igh-J^{tm1Cgn} (B-deficient) BALB/c background mice (Figure 4-6A). These mice were harvested at the early metastatic timepoint of 15 days, which is when metastatic nodules first begin forming in the lungs of the 4T1 orthotopic metastasis model (Figure 4-6A). Routine tumor measurements determined that there was no significant difference in the growth of primary tumors between B-proficient and B-deficient 4T1 orthotopic metastasis models during at 15 days post tumor cell injection (Figure 4-6B). Interestingly, initial H&E stains of metastatic lungs sections suggested that B-deficient mice may exhibit reduced formation of lung metastases (Figure 4-6C). To confirm that the lack of B cells impairs the ability of 4T1 tumors to form lung metastases through a reduction in the invasive ability of tumor cells in B-deficient mice, we stained five lung sections taken at ≥20μm intervals from B-proficient and B-deficient orthotopic metastasis models for cytokeratin-14 (K14) (Figure 4-6F). Studies from the Ewald lab reported that K14 is a marker for invasive leader cells located at the invasive fronts of BC primary tumors, lung metastases, and organoids.[239] Quantification of the average number of metastatic nodules per lung from 5 lung sections sectioned at ≥20μm intervals from each mouse showed that B-deficient 4T1 orthotopic metastasis models had significantly reduced lung metastases, suggesting that the lack of B cells impaired metastatic colonization of the lung (Figure 4-6D). In line with our previous findings that metastasis-infiltrating B cell proportions were higher in smaller micrometastases, we stratified each lung metastasis from B-proficient and B-deficient 4T1 orthotopic metastasis models into micro, medium-, and macrometastases and found that B-deficient mice had a significantly lower number of micrometastases compared to larger metastases (Figure 4-6E).

Based on our data that showed that B cells can promote the invasion and migration of tumor cells *in vitro*, we analyzed the proportion of $K14^+$ tumor cells to total tumor cells in each lung metastasis as a measurement of the number of invasive leader cells and invasive fronts. In line with our *in vitro* assay results, we found that the lung metastases from B-deficient mice had significantly reduced proportions of $K14^+$ tumor cells, which is indicative of a reduction in the number of invasive leader cells and invasive fronts (Figure 4-6F, G). Taken together, our *in vivo* data suggests that B cells promote the development of invasive fronts and invasive leaders cells in lung metastases and the absence of B cells impairs the invasiveness and development of TNBC lung metastases.

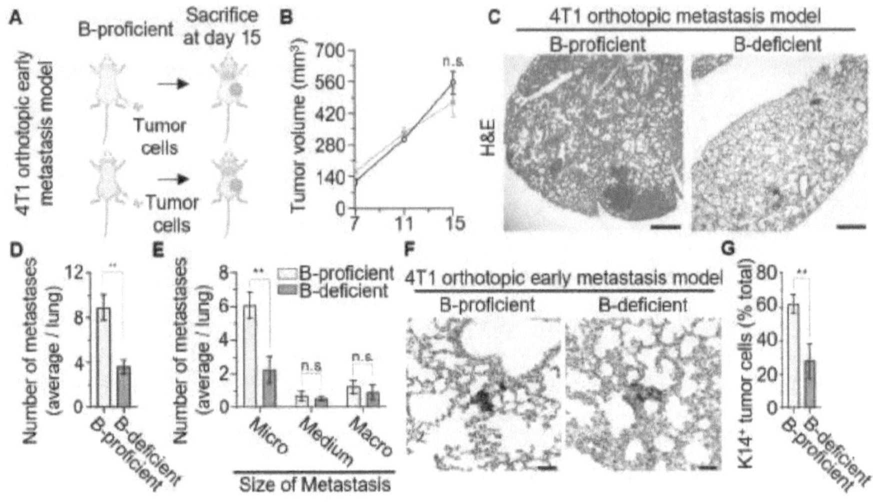

Figure 4-6: B cell-deficient mice show reduced invasive fronts and micrometastases in early orthotopic metastatic disease

(**A**) Schematic depicting the generation of 4T1 orthotopic early metastasis models through injection of 5×10^5 4T1 tumor cells into the fourth mammary gland of 6- to 8-week old female syngeneic BALB/cJ (B-proficient, top) and B cell-deficient Igh-J^{tm1Cgn} (B-deficient, bottom) mice with a BALB/c background. Mice were sacrificed and lungs were collected at the early metastatic timepoint of 15 days post injection. (**B**) Tumor growth in B-proficient and B deficient 4T1 orthotopic early metastasis models. (**C**) Representative images of lung sections from 4T1 B-proficient (left) and B-deficient (right) orthotopic early metastasis models taken at 15 days post tumor-cell injection and stained with hematoxylin and eosin (H&E). Scale bars represents 50μm. (**D**) Bar graphs depicting the average number of lung metastases per lung from 5 lung sections sectioned at $\geq$20μm intervals from B-proficient and B-deficient 4T1 orthotopic early metastasis models. (**E**) Bar graphs depicting the average number of lung micro- (1-50 tumor cells), medium- (51-100 tumor cells), and macrometastases (>100 tumor cells) per lung from 5 lung sections sectioned at $\geq$20μm intervals from B-proficient and B-deficient 4T1 orthotopic early metastasis models. (**G, H**) Representative images of lung sections from B-proficient (left) and B-deficient (right) 4T1 orthotopic early metastasis models taken at 15 days post tumor-cell injection and immunostained using antibodies against K14 for invasive margin tumor cells (**G**). Scale bars represent 50μm. Bar graphs depicting the number of K14[+] invasive margin tumor cells as a proportion of total tumor cells from each lung metastasis from B-proficient and B-deficient 4T1 orthotopic metastasis models (**H**). n = 6-7 mice for B-proficient 4T1 orthotopic metastasis models. n = 4 mice for B-deficient 4T1 orthotopic metastasis models. *n.s.* not significant, * p<0.05, ** p<0.01

4.7 B cells are associated with upregulated tumor cell expression of phosphorylated-mTOR (Ser2448)

To determine upregulated invasion-associated pathways, we performed immunohistochemical staining of metastatic lungs sections from 4T1 B-proficient and B-deficient orthotopic early metastasis models for markers of growth and invasion pathways. Among these pathways, quantitative analysis revealed that that the lung metastases from B-deficient mice had significantly reduced proportions of p-mTOR[+] tumor cells compared to B-proficient mice (Figure 4-7A, B). p-mTOR is constitutively activated and through activation of downstream pathways, has been shown to promote the invasion of TNBC cells; and its expression is associated with tumor cells at invasive fronts and is elevated in metastases when compared to primary tumors.[243-248] To further clinically validate these findings, we stained human TNBC patients, with high or low TIB density determined in a blinded pathological

analysis by an independent pathologist, for p-mTOR (Figure 4-7C). Scoring of lung metastases

for high or low p-mTOR expression revealed that TNBC patient lung metastases with high TIBs

were significantly correlated with high p-mTOR-tumor cell expression compared to TNBC

patients with low TIBs (Figure 4-7D). Taken altogether, our *in vivo* and clinical data suggests

that B cells promote the phosphorylation and activation of mTOR at Ser2448 to promote the

invasion and development of invasive fronts and invasive leader cells in TNBC lung metastases.

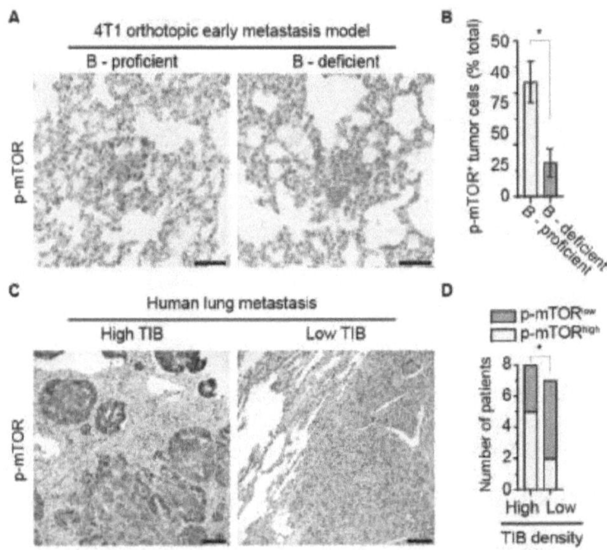

Figure 4-7: B cells are associated with upregulated tumor cell expression of

phosphorylated-mTOR

(**A, B**) Representative images (**A**) of lung sections from B-proficient (left) and B-deficient (right)

4T1 orthotopic early metastasis models taken at 15 days post tumor-cell injection and immunostained using antibodies against p-mTOR (Ser2448). Scale bars represent 50μm. Bar graphs (**B**) depicting the number of p-mTOR⁺ tumor cells as a proportion of total tumor cells from each lung metastasis from B-proficient and B-deficient 4T1 orthotopic early metastasis models. $n = 7$ mice for B-proficient 4T1 orthotopic metastasis models. $n = 4$ mice for B-deficient 4T1 orthotopic metastasis models. (C-D) Representative images (C) of lung sections with high (left) and low (right) tumor-infiltrating B cell (TIB) density from human triple-negative breast cancer patients immunostained with antibodies against p-mTOR (Ser2448). Scale bars represent 100μm. Bar graphs (D) depicting blinded scoring of p-mTOR (Ser2448)-stained lung metastases as high or low p-mTOR expression from TIB high and low human triple-negative breast cancer patients. $n = 8$ TIB high triple-negative breast cancer patients. $n = 7$ TIB low triple-negative breast cancer patients. In panel D, data is expressed as the number of triple-negative breast cancer patients and the p-value was determined using Pearson's chi-squared test. In panel B, data is expressed as mean $\pm$ the standard error of the mean and p-values were determined by the two-tailed, unpaired Student's t-test. * $p<0.05$

4.8 Discussion

The challenges of managing TNBC lies in the lack of effective targeted treatments and the reduction of efficacy in available immunotherapies in metastatic disease. The limited efficacy of treatments for mTNBC suggests that the discovery of novel tumor-promoting mechanisms and revaluation of overlooked cell types is urgently needed. Although B cells have generally been overlooked in tumor immunology due to their canonically accepted role in pro-inflammatory anti-tumor function as APCs or antigen-secreting PCs, there is growing evidence that B cells can function in tumor-promoting roles as well. The discovery of Bregs in the 1970's, which mediate the immunosuppression of anti-tumor responses and T cell function, revealed that specific B cell subsets can function in tumor-promoting roles.[249,250] Although studies elucidating the tumor-promoting roles of B cells remain marginal compared to those on myeloid or T cells, there is growing evidence that prognostic impact and anti- or pro- tumor function of B cells can be dependent on 1) spatial distribution (TLS-B, LC-B, or TIBs) and localization, 2) B cell subtype, such as Bregs and PCs, and 3) their polarization and function.

The mTOR pathway

The elucidation of the mammalian target of rapamycin (mTOR) was the culmination of over three decades of research. In 1964, Ayerst Research Laboratories discovered and isolated an anti-fungal macrolide antibiotic from the soil bacterium, *Strepomyces hygroscopicus*, and named it "rapamycin" after the island where the bacterium was discovered: Rapa Nui, or Easter Island.[251] Initial studies on rapamycin revealed several indications against tumors and roles in immunosuppression, although it's specific mechanism of action remained unknown. In 1990 and 1994, it was finally revealed that rapamycin forms a complex with prolyl-isomerase FKBP12, which then binds to mTOR to inhibit G1 cell-cycle progression and proliferation.[252,253] Subsequent studies on mTOR have further revealed its role as a critical node that integrates with many major and minor signaling pathways to function as a master regulator of cell growth and metabolism.[254]

mTOR is characterized as a 289-kDa serine/threonine protein kinase belonging to the PI3K protein kinase (PIKK) family and is the catalytic subunit of mTOR complexes 1 and 2 (mTORC1/2) through binding with regulatory-associated protein of mTOR (RAPTOR) and rapamycin-insensitive companion of mTOR (RICTOR) scaffolding proteins, respectively.[254] mTORC1 functions as a regulator that integrates upstream signaling, nutritional, and stress information to promote downstream biosynthesis, cell metabolism and catabolism, autophagy, and cell growth through phosphorylation of downstream effectors, such as ribosomal p70 S6 kinase (p70S6K) and eukaryotic translation initiation factor 4E (4E-BP1). Phosphorylation by mTORC1 at Thr389 activates p70S6K, which then upregulates protein and nucleotide synthesis. Phosphorylation inhibits 4E-BP1, which is a negative regulator of 5' cap-dependent mRNA translation, to promote protein synthesis. Specifically, extracellular positive upstream regulators of mTORC1 signaling include ample supplies of oxygen, amino acids, lipids, and growth/mitogen/cytokine factor signaling (such as TGF-β, TNF-α, insulin, and IGF) which activates RAS/ERK, PI3K, AKT, and IKKβ signaling pathways that inhibit TSC, a negative regulator "brake" for mTORC1 activity, through phosphorylation of its TSC2 subunit. TSC functions as a GTPase-activating protein that inhibits Rag and Rheb GTPase G proteins by catalyzing their active GTP-bound states to inactive GDP-bound states. Activated GTP-bound RAG conditionally recruits and anchors mTORC1 to lysosomes in the presence of abundant intracellular amino acids, glucose, and other nutrients. Activated GTP-bound Rheb then conditionally activates the RAG-bound mTORC1 upon inhibition of TSC from upstream signaling pathways. Conversely, nutrient deprivation, energetic stress, hypoxia, and the p53/PTEN-mediated DNA damage pathways activate TSC to inhibit mTORC1 activity.[254]

mTORC2 integrates upstream information from signaling pathways to control downstream cytoskeleton remodeling and cell survival and proliferation through activation and phosphorylation of AKT, protein kinase C α, focal adhesion proteins and small GTPase Rho and Rac proteins.[254,255] mTORC2 is primarily activated by growth factor and insulin signaling through Ras, AKT, and PI3K signaling pathways and inhibited in the absence of insulin. Furthermore, activated mTORC1 forms a negative-feedback loop to downregulate the insulin/PI3K/AKT pathway to inhibit mTORC2. Interestingly, mTORC1 is strongly inhibited even by acute rapamycin treatment while inhibition of mTORC2 requires prolonged chronic rapamycin treatment.[254]

mTOR, as a serine/threonine kinase, contains a multitude of phosphorylation sites that promotes its activation: mTOCR1 only (Ser1415, Ser2159, Thr2164, and Thr2446); mTORC1/2 (Ser1261, Ser2448, and Ser2481).[256] Specifically, phosphorylation of mTOR Ser2448 (from here on, abbreviated as p-mTOR) renders mTOR constitutively active and is implicated in a multitude of diseases. p-mTOR phosphorylation is mediated by a positive feedback loop in which activated mTOR phosphorylates and activates S70S6K, which then phosphorylates mTOR at Ser2448.[257] Therefore, p-mTOR functions as a positive feedback loop upon initial activation of mTOR.

p-mTOR in triple-negative breast cancer and invasion

Because of its integration with cellular pathways that are often mutated or dysregulated in cancer cells and its central role in regulating cellular metabolism, cytoskeleton remodeling, growth, survival, and proliferation, mTOR activity is frequently upregulated, phosphorylated, and has a broad range of implications in many cancer types, including TNBC. Interestingly, p-mTOR expression was found to be not only upregulated in cancer tissues, but invading leader cells (lung cancer, CRC and PDAC) and metastases (renal cell carcinoma and hepatocellular carcinoma) had the higher p-mTOR expression compared to primary tumors, suggesting that p-mTOR and it's downstream pathways play an important functional role in metastasis and invasion.[244] Clinical studies on human BC patients have revealed that AKT, mTOR, p-mTOR, and downstream p-p70S6K and p-4E-BP1 pathways are aberrantly activated upon transition from normal breast epithelium to ductal carcinoma in situ and invasive BC.[258,259] Furthermore the studies found that

72% of TNBC tumors were p-mTOR[+] and patients with p-mTOR[+] or mTOR overexpression BC, including TNBC, had significantly worse overall and recurrence-free survival (RFS).[258,260] Interestingly, p-mTOR, p-p70S6K, and p-4E-BP1 were found to be associated with HER2-positive BCs and *in vitro* transwell studies have shown that overexpressing HER2 in HER[-] BC cell lines, 435.eB (TNBC) and MCF7.eB (luminal), had higher p-mTOR and p-4E-BP1 expression and increased invasion compared to their parental HER2[-] cell lines, MDA-MB-435 and MCF7.[243] Another clinical study revealed the high mTOR and p-mTOR expression is significantly associated with TNBCs compared to other BC subtypes.[261] Furthermore, another study revealed through active kinase and pharmacological profiling that mTOR inhibitors demonstrated elevated efficacy in inhibiting the proliferation of TNBC cell lines and tumor growth in TNBC mouse models.[262]

Indeed, studies have uncovered numerous mechanisms on how mTORC1 activity and downstream mediators can promote cell migration and invasion. Rapamycin treatment was found to inhibit the migration of IGF-stimulated TNBC MDA-MB-468 cell lines (along with other cancer cell lines) through inhibition of mTORC1 mediated phosphorylation of p70S6K and 4E-BP1.[263] Additional studies showed that activated mTOR, p60S6K, and AKT are localized to the actin arc at the leading edge of actively migrating Swiss 3T3 cells and treatment with rapamycin blocked actin arc formation.[255] Furthermore, mTORC1 activation was found to induce the expression of FSCN1, an actin-bundling protein that promotes migration and metastasis in cancers, in CRC HT-29 cells and treatment of HT-29 cells with mTOR inhibitors, everolimus or rapamycin, inhibited mTORC1 activation, suppressed FSCN1 expression, and reduced tumor cell motility and proliferation.[264,265] Another study revealed that TGF-β/SMAD signaling-induced mTOR activation and phosphorylation of p70S6K and 4E-BP1 mediates EMT and increased cell size in the NMugMG murine mammary epithelial cell line.[266] p70S6K has also been shown to promote phosphorylation of focal adhesion proteins, such as FAK, and remodeling of F-actin for the formation of lamellipodia to facilitate invasion of multiple cancer cell lines.[267]

Another potential mechanism of mTOR-mediated promotion of TNBC invasion is through hypoxia-inducible factor 1 (HIF1α). Although HIF1α expression can be induced independently from mTORC1 activity, active mTORC1 is sufficient to activate HIF1α, a transcription factor, through suppression of 4E-BP1 activity, which activates 5' cap-dependent mRNA translation of the 5' untranslated region of HI1Fα mRNA.[245] HIF1α is found to be hyperactivated in multiple basal-like tumors, including TNBC with the highest expression in invasive leader cells, and is associated with poor prognosis, reduced RFS, EMT (transcriptional control of E-cadherin, SNAIL, ZEB1, and TWIST), angiogenesis (upregulation of VEGFA) radio and chemotherapy resistance, increased invasion (transcriptional activation of CSRP2, an invadopodia actin bundling protein that induces the formation of invadopodia), and metastasis.[245-248] In addition to cell-intrinsic promotion of motility, activation of mTOR and downstream effectors, including HIF1α) has also been shown to promote the expression of ECM remodeling proteins, such as MMP-2/9 and uPA, which function in breaking down ECM components to help facilitate cell invasion through the ECM.[255] A recent study also revealed that treatment of TNBC MDA-MB-231 and MCF7 cell lines with Berbamine downregulated the PI3K/AKT/mTOR pathway and reduced tumor cell invasion *in vitro*.[268] Another study showed that knockdown of TSC in the TSC^KO MMTV-PyMT GEMM of BC hyperactivated mTORC1, which induced AKT signaling and resulted in accelerated tumor growth, and lung metastasis *in vivo* and increased *in vitro* invasion using transwell invasion assays.[269]

Although less studied than mTORC1, mTORC2 has also been shown to promote cell migration and invasion through regulation of downstream Rho/Rac-GTPases that in turn, regulate actin cytoskeleton restructuring. Knockdown of mTOR or RICTOR in HEK293 or 3T3 fibroblast cells was found to inhibit the polymerization of actin, the formation of lamellipodia, and cell spreading and migration.[270] Furthermore, inhibition of RICTOR in several BC and TNBC cell lines, MDA-MB-231, MDA-MB-468, BT549 and MCF7, inhibited TGF-β-mediated mTOR-RICTOR-ILK (integrin linked kinase) function and blocked EMT and invasion.[271] Taken together, these studies indicate that activated mTOR or p-mTOR and downstream effectors are integrally linked to tumor cell motility and invasion.[263]

Key findings

Here, we present evidence in both human mTNBC patients and multiple murine TNBC orthotopic and experimental metastasis that there is a population of B220$^+$ B cells that are recruited specifically to the invasive margin of TNBC lung metastases. Furthermore, we show that lung B cells from TNBC mouse models directly promote the invasion and migration of TNBC lung metastasis-derived organoids and cell lines, respectively, in co-culture. Interestingly, because peripheral B cells from TNBC mouse models also enhanced lung metastasis-organoid invasion in co-culture and that B cells kept in proximity, but not directly touching, to tumor cells still enhanced tumor cell migration, the data suggests that B cells can be "educated" via a paracrine signaling mechanism by tumor cells to promote tumor cell motility through secreted factors. It is important to distinguish that promotion of invasion within a 3D microenvironment, such as a Matrigel matrix, could also be caused by ECM degradation and remodeling, as has been shown with tumor-associated myeloid cells.[81] However, the transwell migration assay did not utilize an ECM matrix to evaluate migration, which suggests that the B cell-secreted factor that promotes tumor cell invasion and migration directly affects the tumor cell itself and not it's microenvironment.

Furthermore, we validated *in vivo* that B-deficient mice exhibit impaired formation of lung metastasis along with a concomitant reduction in the number of K14[+] invasive leader tumor cells and p-mTOR[+] tumor cells in their lung metastases during early metastatic progression. This suggests that a B cell-derived factor induces the phosphorylation of p-mTOR at Ser2448, which can promote tumor cell invasion through downstream pathways and that while B cell-mediated invasion promotion through p-mTOR may not be required for the formation of lung metastasis, the mechanism does play a role in promoting the invasion and development of TNBC lung metastases during early metastatic colonization. This data is consistent with studies showing that 1) mTOR/p-mTOR expression is highest in invading leader tumor cells and metastases[244], 2) patients with p-mTOR[+] TNBC have significantly poorer RFS[258,260], and 3) that the mTOR/p-mTOR pathways can promote invasion through a variety of downstream mechanisms, such as induction of EMT[266] and action/cytoskeleton remodeling and formation of lamellipodia and invadopodia.[246,255]

Interestingly, metastasis-infiltrating B cell density was found to highest in smaller micrometastases, which correlated with the observation that the reduction of lung metastases in B-deficient was primarily in micrometastases. Because mTOR lies at the nexus of many metabolic, nutrition, and growth factor signaling pathways and the phosphorylation of mTOR at Ser2448 is mediated in a positive feedback loop from downstream p70S6K, it is possible the B-cell mediated p-mTOR and downstream invasion-promoting mechanisms may be redundant with other non-tumor cells in the TME. In this scenario, B cells are not required for the formation of lung metastases, but instead provide additional tumor-promoting support to micrometastases through p-mTOR until other tumor-promoting cells are recruited into the TME with functionally redundant roles in mTOR phosphorylation and invasion-promotion. Indeed, while there are many B cell-secreted factors that can activate mTOR (IL-2[272], IL-4[273], IL-6[274], IL-12[275], TGF-β[276], and TNF-α[277]), these factors can also be secreted by other cell types in the TME. Additionally, mTOR can also be activated by a host of other non B cell-secreted factors (IL-1[278], IL-13[279], IL-27[280], IGF-1[263,281], VEGF[282], and PDGF[283]). Regardless, taken together, our findings suggest that the putative p-mTOR-mediated invasion-promotion of tumor cells by B cells on small micrometastases may present a novel therapeutic option for advanced or mTNBC patients and TNBC patients with RCB. Therapeutic blockade of either B cell recruitment into the TME or mTOR/p-mTOR could delay or prevent small micrometastases in patients with RCB from relapsing.

Study limitations

There are several limitations to our findings. The first is the phenotyping of metastasis-infiltrating tumor-educated B cells. Another is elucidating the signaling mechanism mediating tumor cell-B cell crosstalk and coupling the paracrine signaling axis to p-mTOR and downstream mediators of invasion. Furthermore, *in vitro* and *in vivo* functional assays using mTOR inhibitors or knockdown of mTOR-associated components will need to be performed to validate the role of p-mTOR in mediating invasion and lung metastasis. The strategy and experimental designs for addressing these limitations are described in the following sections.

However, there is a study that, at a glance, may contradict our findings. Wortman and colleagues recently revealed in a retrospective clinical study that increased number of spatially dispersed CD20$^+$ B cells as either single TIBs or LC-Bs within tumor nests in primary tumors are associated with improved RFS and good prognosis in TNBC patients.[93] This suggests that TIBs in primary TNBC tumors function in an anti-tumor role. However, the study has several limitations as well. Firstly, they did not assess the phenotype or function of these TIBs. Second, the study analyzed a small cohort of 36 TNBC patients with differing disease characteristics and non-uniform treatment regiments.[93] Therefore, their findings that associate pre-treatment TIBs to post-treatment RFS can be confounded by these factors. There are also many other factors that de-couple their findings from our study. Firstly, Wortman and colleagues did not analyze TIBs at the invasive margin between the primary tumor and breast tissue. Although they did differentiate stromal TIBs from tumor nest TIBs, these TIBs are still intratumoral TIBs and not located at the invasive margin between the primary tumor and breast tissue. Given that spatial localization can determine the function and phenotype of immune cells and that p-mTOR expression is higher in tumor cells at the invasive margin, it is plausible that the invasive margin-localized TIBs in our study are functionally distinct from the TIBs analyzed.[244] Furthermore, tumor cells between primary tumors and their metastases are distinct, as tumor cells need to adopt organ-specific programs to form metastatic colonies.[18] These organ-specific programs could alter the intrinsic properties of metastasized tumor cells, which can affect their interaction and signaling with immune cells. Indeed, there are studies showing that immune populations, signaling pathways, and TME composition between matched BC primary tumors and their metastases are distinct from one another.[71,284,285] Furthermore, we show that lung metastases can recruit B cells to their invasive margin independent of a primary tumor and that 4T1 B-deficient models exhibit no differences in primary tumor growth but impaired development of lung metastases compared B-proficient models. Taken together, these differences suggests that the anti-tumor TIBs proposed by Wortman and colleagues are functionally different from the invasion-promoting, invasive margin-localized, metastasis-infiltrating B cells we report in our study. One limitation to this conclusion is that we also report that B cells can be educated in co-culture with 4T1 cells lines to promote migration. However, an explanation for this discrepancy is that our co-culture assay only utilized tumor cells and B cells and was devoid of other heterogenous interactions with other cell types and signaling pathways that may be found in the TME of primary tumors, which are distinct from metastasis-associated TME, that may polarize B cells toward an anti-tumor function. Taken altogether, despite somewhat conflicting results from Wortmann and colleagues, there are many discrepancies and differences between their study parameters and ours, which suggests that their results need to be considered as separate and distinct entities that are taken in a different context.

Future perspectives: Elucidating the invasion-promoting B cell-tumor cell-p-mTOR axis

Further studies are needed to dissect the precise signaling mechanisms between tumor cell-B cell crosstalk and to evaluate the efficacy of inhibitors on this invasion-promoting mechanism. To determine whether B cell-secreted factors activate and phosphorylate mTOR in tumor cells to promote invasion, RT-qPCR and immunoblots are needed to confirm the upregulated tumor cell-phosphorylation of mTOR at Ser2448 in tumor cell-B cell co-culture. Furthermore, mTOR inhibitors, such as rapamycin or everolimus, can be added into tumor cell-B cell coculture to test if inhibition of mTOR blocks B cell-mediated tumor cell invasion promotion. To identify candidate B cell-secreted factors mediating mTOR activation in tumor cells, proteomic strategies, such as mass spectrometry, ELISA, or protein microarrays, can be utilized to test the conditioned media taken from tumor cells co-cultured with B cells for B cell-secreted factors known to activate or phosphorylate mTOR. Following this, specific inhibitors targeting candidate B cell-secreted factors can be evaluated and screened for using the co-culture invasion assay system. However, if B cell-mediated tumor cell-mTOR activation is functionally redundant to other signaling pathways mediated by other cell types, then it may be more strategically feasible to direct efforts into inhibiting tumor-mTOR/p-mTOR or downstream targets, such as p70S6K, AKT, and HIF1α, mediators of EMT, and mediators of actin/cytoskeleton remodeling. The expression and function of these downstream targets can be evaluated through RT-qPCR or immunoblotting of tumor cells co-cultured with B cells and with or without treatment by mTOR inhibitors. Mediators of the B cell-tumor cell-mTOR invasion promoting pathway can then be validated *in vivo* by treating 4T1 orthotopic early metastasis models with inhibitors targeting mTOR/p-mTOR or upstream and downstream effectors.

Preclinical BC mouse models have demonstrated the efficacy of targeting mTOR/mTORC1/2 in a metastatic and invasion context. One study revealed that conditional knockout or suppression of RICTOR in HER2[+] BC models using RICTOR[FL/FL] MMTV-NIC mice or orthotopic and experimental metastasis models using MDA-MB-361 expressing RICTOR shRNA exhibited reduced lung metastasis through loss of RICTOR-dependent RAC1-mediated invasion.[286] Other studies show that treatment of seven TNBC patient-derived xenograft mouse models with rapamycin resulted in 77-99% reduction in tumor growth, and inhibiting mTOR/p-mTOR in multiple BC and TNBC cell lines and mouse models through either rapamycin alone or combined with MLN8237 (Aurora-A inhibitor, upstream of mTOR signaling) reduced tumor cell proliferation and migration *in vitro* and reduced tumor growth *in vivo*. [287,288] Although these studies showed there was no complete tumor regression nor analyzed the effects of mTOR inhibition on metastasis[287,288], another study revealed that treatment of TNBC xenograft MDA-MB-231 LM2 experimental metastasis models with everolimus significantly reduced lung metastasis.[289]

There are a limited number of studies targeting mTOR using the 4T1 TNBC orthotopic metastasis model. One of these demonstrated that additional treatment of doxorubicin-treated 4T1 TNBC orthotopic metastasis models with metformin further reduced tumor growth compared to doxorubicin alone through inhibition of the AKT/STAT3/mTOR pathway.[290] However, the study did not analyze the effects of metformin-associated inhibition of mTOR on lung metastasis. A recent study revealed that 4T1 lung metastases have elevated expression of mTORC1 compared to matched primary tumors and targeting mTORC1 expression via inhibiting upstream the serine biosynthesis pathway through targeting MCT2 (pyruvate uptake) and silencing *PHGDH* reduced primary tumor growth and the development of lung metastasis.[291] The study did not analyze mediators of invasion downstream of mTORC1, however, it does provide an example of a redundant pathway in which 4T1 cells can activate mTOR to promote lung metastasis. Interestingly, there is one study that showed that treatment of 4T1 orthotopic metastasis models after surgical resection with rapamycin increased lung metastasis through rapamycin-induced expansion of immunosuppressive Tregs.[292] However, it should also be noted that acute rapamycin treatment does not affect mTORC2, which studies show can also mediate tumor invasion, and further testing with pan-mTORC1/2 inhibitors, such as AZD2014, should be utilized. Furthermore, there are other studies that show that 1) combination treatment using the PI3K/mTOR inhibitor, gedatolisib, with ICIs significantly reduced tumor growth and increased tumor-infiltrating CTLs in luminal/triple-negative-like PyMT BC orthotopic mouse models; and 2) combination treatment using the mTORC1/2 inhibitor, AZD2014, with ICIs reduced tumor-infiltrating Tregs and reduced tumor growth and improved survival in MC38 and CT-26 mouse models of colon cancer.[293] These studies suggest that mTOR-inhibition-induced immunosuppression can be abrogated with the application of combination treatment.[293]

However, another complication to mTOR inhibition is the acquisition of resistance. Mateo and colleagues showed that prolonged inhibition of mTOR in BC MCF7 and TNBC HCC1937 cell lines and 4T1 orthotopic models with everolimus induced a feedback mechanism that upregulated the expression of *EVI1* and *SOX9*.[289] This resulted in the upregulation of upstream promoters of mTOR activity, *RAPTOR* and *RHEB*, and *FSCN1*, a downstream mTOR-associated mediator of actin remodeling associated with invasion and metastasis, and no reduction in lung metastasis.[289] Furthermore, depletion of EVI1, SOX9, or FSCN1 in 4T1 or MDA-MB-231 LM2 was found to significantly impair the formation lung metastasis *in vivo*.[289] Other mechanisms of mTOR inhibitor resistance include the emergence and selection for clonal populations that have acquired mutations in mTOR kinase domains or mTOR-associated FKBP12.[294] This suggests that in addition to mTOR-induced immunosuppression; acquisition of resistance is another complication associated with monotreatment with mTOR inhibitors. However, mTOR inhibition used in a neoadjuvant setting to delay or prevent relapse from RCB may still prove to be efficacious. Furthermore, third generation mTOR inhibitors, such as rapalink-1, a conjugate drug of two mTOR inhibitors, rapamycin and MLN0128, have been shown to overcome mTOR resistance mutations in mTOR-resistant MCF-7 BC cell lines treated with first and second generation mTOR inhibitors.[294] Additional studies have shown that rapalink-1 is well tolerated and demonstrates enhanced *in vitro* and *in vivo* tumor-suppressive effects on multiple sunitinib-(a receptor tyrosine kinase inhibitor) resistant cell lines and mouse models of renal cell carcinoma compared to temosirolimus.[295] Taken together, these studies suggest that mTOR inhibition, in combination with other anti-tumor agents or usage of improved third generation mTOR inhibitors, can be utilized in preclinical mouse models of TNBC to investigate the invasion-promoting mechanisms of the B cell-tumor cell-p-mTOR reported here and to evaluate their efficacy in a neoadjuvant setting to delay relapse from RCB in surgically-resected models.

Future perspectives: Targeting mTOR or B cells in breast cancer patients

Currently, only everolimus, a second generation mTOR kinase inhibitor, is approved in combination with exemestane, an aromatase inhibitor, for the treatment BC patients, albeit for advanced HR$^+$ HER2$^-$ BC patients. [296,297] The combination treatment was found to extend mPFS and mOS to 6.9 months and 10.6 months compared to 2.8 months and 4.1 months, respectively, with placebo and exemestane treatment.[296,297] The phase II clinical trial, NCT01127763, found that everolimus in combination with carboplatin in TNBC resulted in a clinical benefit rate of 36% with mPFS and OS of 3 months and 16.6 months.[298] However, another mTOR inhibitor, temsirolimus, exhibited no response from TNBC patients in the phase II clinical trial,NCT01111825.[299] Other clinical trials are currently testing other mTOR inhibitors, such as AZD2014[300,301] and PQR309[302], which could be additional promising agents to test in our models. Interestingly, studies have shown that monotherapy with mTOR inhibitors resulted in acquisition of resistance and no clinical benefit through elevated phosphorylated-AKT due to a negative feedback loop, thusly necessitating that mTOR inhibitors be combined with other chemotherapeutic agents.[303] This is consistent with our findings that B cell-deficient mice, while exhibiting reduced p-mTOR expression and invasive leader cells in their lung metastases, were still able to develop lung metastasis. However, while mTOR inhibitiors may not be efficacious as monotherapies, they may be still provide clinical benefit when combined with other anti-cancer agents and our findings suggest that inhibition of mTOR may be useful in a neoadjuvant setting to treat TNBC patients with RCB to prevent or delay relapse. This strategy can be tested in preclinical TNBC orthotopic mouse models through timed surgical resection of the primary tumor and treatment with mTOR inhibitors, followed by bioluminescent imaging to detect RCB, metastasis, and relapse.

Another therapeutic strategy may be to target metastasis-infiltrating B cells. Although B-deficient mice show impaired formation of TNBC lung metastasis, it may not be viable to deplete all B cell subsets when evaluating therapeutic options as they can deplete anti-tumor B cells in addition to tumor-promoting B cell subsets. Furthermore, studies have shown that treatment of preclinical BC EMT6 and 4T1.2 mouse models with an anti-CD20 antibody depleted most B cell populations, but enriched for CD20[low] and CD19[+] Bregs, which resulted in increased Treg and enhanced tumor growth and lung metastasis.[125,126] Currently, there are no approved B cell immunotherapies for the treatment of TNBC patients. The BTK inhibitor, Ibruitinib, which targets B cell BCR signaling and inhibits MDSC formation, had shown promising results in preclinical mouse models of TNBC, but poor ORR (3%) in mTNBC patients.[85-88] These findings suggest that specific depletion of tumor-promoting B cell subsets may be a superior strategy compared to pan-B cell depletion.

Future perspectives: Elucidating the phenotype of tumor-infiltrating B cells

However, there are significant challenges in elucidating the specific subset of metastasis-infiltrating, tumor-educated B cells. Some studies have shown that co-culturing B cells with PD-L1[hi] human TNBC MDA-MB-231 or murine TNBC 4T1 and 4T1.2 cell lines induced Breg differentiation.[120,123] However, these Bregs were found to function in an immunosuppressive role through secretion of IL-10 and induction of Treg differentiation.[123] Furthermore, contradictory results from recent single-cell RNA sequencing and antigen receptor profiling of TIBs cells in TNBC patient tumors revealed that TNBC TIBs were predominantly mature and memory B cell subsets, with a lack of any significant IL10[+] Breg populations.[304] However, these studies were primarily conducted in either *in vitro* cell culture (former) or using primary tumor samples (latter) and not using metastasis-derived cells or in a metastatic context. Further studies are needed to identify the phenotype or subtype of invasion-promoting metastasis-infiltrating B cells.

There are several challenges to anticipate when phenotyping these metastasis-infiltrating B cells. Firstly, if proximity and spatial localization is critical for this specific B cell phenotype, then flow cytometry on whole metastatic lungs may not be sensitive enough to detect such a small population – as non tumor-infiltrating B cells in the lungs may be the predominant population. Flow cytometry also would be unable to determine spatial localization and additional tissue preparation steps may be needed to enrich for lung metastases. One such technique would be laser capture microdissection techniques to isolate lung metastases, however there may issues with epitope degradation using fixed tissues.[305] In addition, the B cells may lose their tumor-educated phenotype if removed from the proximity of lung metastases. Therefore, our *ex vivo* 3D organoid co-culture system may represent a useful model for the phenotyping of metastasis-infiltrating B cells. Taken together, our findings show that further elucidation of the phenotype of metastasis-infiltrating B cells and targeting mTOR/p-mTOR and its downstream invasion-promoting pathways may provide efficacious therapeutic targets for the treatment of mTNBC patients and TNBC patients with RCB.

Conclusions and future directions

Stage IV metastatic cancers generally represent an incurable and terminal illness that is causative of about 90% of all cancer-associated mortality.[4] As a cancer progresses toward and develops metastatic disease, interactions between tumor cells and non-tumor cells causes the release of soluble factors, exosomes, and metabolites that systemically and detrimentally alter host physiology, metabolism, and immune regulation.[133] This physiological reprogramming often culminates in cachexia and aberrant tumor-promoting immune cell phenotypes.[153]

Our studies on metastatic PDAC- and BRCA-like TNBC-associated cachexia demonstrates that upregulation of muscle-cell ZIP14 expression along with concomitant increase in intramuscular zinc ion levels is directly correlated to the development of cachexia. This data is consistent with our previous findings that the ZIP14-zinc axis mediates cachexia development in metastatic mouse models of breast, lung, and colon cancer.[171] The previous study also showed that muscle-cell expression of ZIP14 is induced by tumor-associated TGF-β and TNF-α.[171] Taken together, these findings suggest that targeting either upstream mediators of muscle-cell ZIP14 expression or ZIP14 blockade and zinc chelation strategies should be tested in preclinical metastatic mouse models of cachexia to determine potential strategies to prevent or treat cancer-associated cachexia.

Our studies also revealed that B220$^+$ B cells are preferentially recruited to the invasive margin of lung metastases from human mTNBC patients and 4T1 and LM3 metastatic mouse models of TNBC. We further demonstrate that B220$^+$ B cells taken from the lungs and blood of mTNBC mouse models enhance the invasion of lung metastasis-derived organoids when co-cultured together. Furthermore, B220$^+$ B cells isolated from the lungs of mTNBC mouse models promoted the migration of TNBC cell lines. These findings suggest that B cell can be educated by crosstalk with TNBC tumor cells into a phenotype that directly promotes the tumor cell invasion and migration. We validated these findings *in vivo* by showing that B-deficient mice exhibited impaired formation of lung metastases concomitant with a reduced proportion of K14$^+$ invasive leader tumor cells and reduced proportion of p-mTOR$^+$ tumor cells in their lung metastases. We further show that the lung metastases of triple-negative breast cancer patients with high tumor-infiltrating B cell density exhibit increased p-mTOR expression compared to patients with low tumor-infiltrating B cell density. These findings suggest that B cells may induce the phosphorylation of mTOR in tumor cells to promote invasion. Interestingly B cell density was found to be highest in micrometastases, which correlated with *in vivo* analysis that showed that the reduction of lung metastases in B-deficient mice was predominantly in the number of micrometastases. Taken altogether, these findings suggest that further studies are needed to dissect the B cell-tumor cell-p-mTOR invasion-promoting signaling axis and to determine the specific phenotype of these metastasis-infiltrating tumor-associated B cells to identify potential therapeutic targets that can help prevent relapse from RCB or treat lung metastases in TNBC patients.

Materials and Methods

Chapter 2

Cell lines

The Pan02 mouse pancreatic adenocarcinoma cell line was derived from a 3-methylcholanthrene carcinogen-induced pancreatic tumor that developed in a C57CL/6 mouse and was purchased from the National Cancer Institute Cell Repository, MD, USA. The FC1242 mouse pancreatic adenocarcinoma cell line was derived from a pancreatic tumor that developed from a $Kras^{+/LSL-G12D}$, $Trp53^{+/LSL-R172H}$, $Pdx1^{Cre}$ GEMM in the Tuveson laboratory (Cold Spring Harbor Laboratory, Cold Spring Harbor, NY, USA). The FC1242 cell line was procured from the Miller laboratory (New York University, New York, NY, USA). Pan02 and FC1242 cell lines were cultured in DMEM supplemented with 10% fetal bovine serum (Sigma, St. Louis, MO, USA), and 1% penicillin/streptomycin (Life Technologies, Carlsbad, CA, USA) and grown in a 37°C humidified incubator with 5% CO_2.

Mouse studies

All mouse studies, experiments, and protocols were approved by The Columbia University Institutional Animal Care and Use Committee (IACUC) and are compliant with ethical guidelines and regulations from the Institute of Comparative Medicine (ICM) at Columbia University Irving Medical Center (CUIMC) with the IACUC-approved protocol: AAAR6450. All mice were housed in CUIMC's pathogen-free barrier facility and fed on Labdiet 5053 (standard diet). Male, 8- to 9-week old C57BL/6 and athymic nude mice were purchased from Jackson laboratory (Bar Harbor, ME, USA) and Envigo (Somerset, NJ, USA), respectively. C57BL/6 and athymic nude mice were injected with 1 x 10^5 murine FC1242 and Pan02 pancreatic adenocarcinoma cells, respectively, into arterial circulation via intra-cardiac injection. Cachexia development was assessed by mouse body condition, monitored using a body-condition scoring system as previously described,[306] and by routine measurements of body weight, hind-limb grip strength, histological and morphometric analysis of muscle sections, and analysis of muscle atrophy-associated molecular markers.

Measurement of body weight and hind-limb grip strength

Measurements of body weight from healthy control mice and Pan02 and FC1242 experimental metastasis models were performed weekly using a bench-top digital balance. All body weight measurements were normalized to the body weight on the day of tumor cell injection (day 0 post injection). Measurements of hind-limb grip strength were taken weekly using a grip strength meter (Columbus Instruments, Columbia, OH, USA). A minimum of five measurements were performed per mouse weekly and the mean values were calculated. The percent grip strength was normalized to the mean initial grip strength values (100%) on the day of tumor cell injection.

Tissue Collection

Gastrocnemius and diaphragm muscles were harvested and fixed in 4% paraformaldehyde for 24 hours at 4°C or snap frozen in liquid nitrogen at stored at -80°C for histological analysis and molecular analysis, respectively. Liver and lung tissues were harvested and fixed in 4% paraformaldehyde for 24 hours at 4°C. All paraformaldehyde-fixed tissues were washed in PBS for an hour and stored in 70% ethanol until further histological processing and analysis.

Histological analysis of metastases and muscle fibers

For histological analysis, paraformaldehyde-fixed paraffin-embedded gastrocnemius, diaphragm, liver, and lung tissues were sectioned at 5µm-thickness onto positive-charged slides and stained with hematoxylin and eosin (H&E). H&E-stained gastrocnemius and diaphragm tissue sections were visualized and imaged using an Eclipse Ni-U microscope (Nikon Corporation,

Tokyo, Japan). H&E-stained liver and lung tissue sections were visualized and imaged under a DM5500B microscope (Leica Microsystems, Wetzlar, Germany).

Analysis of muscle cross-sectional area

Random two or three fields per H&E-stained paraformaldehyde-fixed paraffin-embedded 5µm-thick cross-sections of gastrocnemius muscles were imaged at 20x magnification using a DM5500B microscope (Leica Microsystems, Wetzlar, Germany). Muscle fiber cross-sectional area was quantified using the drawing module in ImageJ (ImageJ software, Version 1.52h, National Institutes of Health, Bethesda, MD, USA) to trace individual muscle fiber boundaries. Muscle fiber cross-sectional areas from tumor-bearing and control mice were stratified by cross-sectional area ranges of various sizes and the percentage of fibers in each range were calculated. The means of cross-sectional areas for each range were determined from replicate muscle samples.

RT-qPCR analysis of gene expression

Snap frozen gastrocnemius and diaphragm muscles were minced into ~1-2mm pieces and 15mg, representative of each sample, were taken from each muscle for total RNA extraction using Trizol (Life Technologies, Carlsbad, CA, USA). Muscle samples were lysed using 5mm steel beads (Qiagen, Hilden, Germany) and the TissueLyser II (Qiagen, Hilden, Germany) instrument. Samples were centrifuged at 18,000 x g for 5 min and the supernatant was isolated and processed using the RNeasy Mini Kit (Qiagen, Hilden, Germany) with DNase treatment while in-column, accounting to manufacturer's instructions. The total purified RNA in each sample was quantified using a Nanodrop spectrophotometer (Thermo Fisher Scientific, Walthom, MA, USA) and 500ng of RNA was reverse transcribed into cDNA using the cDNA Synthesis Kit (Applied Biosystems, Thermo Fisher Scientific, Walthom, MA, USA). RT-qPCR was performed using 10ng of cDNA from each sample mixed with gene-specific primers and SYBR Green PCR master mix (Applied

Biosystems, Thermo Fisher Scientific, Walthom, MA, USA). Primers for *Gapdh* were used as an internal control. RT-qPCR data were analyzed on an Applied Biosystems 7500 Real Time PCR system (Applied Biosystems, Thermo Fisher Scientific, Walthom, MA, USA) and the fold change in gene expression was determined using the $2^{-\Delta\Delta Ct}$ method.[307] RT-qPCR primer sequences used in this study are shown in Table S1.

Table S1: Primers used for qRT-PCR analysis

Name of Gene	Forward primer (5' – 3')	Reverse primer (5' – 3')
Mouse-*Zip14*	GTGTCTCACTGATTAACCTGGC	AGAGCAGCGTTCCAATGGAC
Mouse-*Trim63/MuRF1*	GTGTGAGGTGCCTACTTGCTC	GCTCAGTCTTCTGTCCTTGGA
Mouse-*MAFbx/Fbxo32*	CAGCTTCGTGAGCGACCTC	GGCAGTCGAGAAGTCCAGTC
Mouse-*Fbxo31*	CATGCGGTTCAAGCCACTG	GTCTGGTTACACTTGGTGGAG
Mouse-*Musa1/Fbxo30*	TCGTGGAATGGTAATCTTGC	CCTCCCGTTTCTCTATCACG
Mouse -*Mt1*	AAGAGTGAGTTGGGACACCT	CGAGACAATACAATGGCCTCC
Mouse -*Mt2*	GCCTGCAAATGCAAACAATGC	AGCTGCACTTGTCGGAAGC
Mouse - *Gapdh*	AGGTCGGTGTGAACGGATTTG	TGTAGACCATGTAGTTGAGGTCA

Table S1: Sequences of primers used in the study for gene expression analysis of murine *Zip14*, *Trim63/MuRF1*, *MAFBx/Fbxo32*, *Fbxo31*, *Musa1/Fbxo30*, *Mt1*, *Mt2* and *Gapdh*

Intramuscular metal ion analysis

15-20mg of each gastrocnemius muscle were sent to the Veterinary Diagnostic Laboratory at Michigan State University, MI, USA, for metal ion analysis. Tissues were dried overnight at 75°C, digested overnight in 10x volume relative to muscle dry weight of nitric acid, and diluted in a 100-fold volume of water. Inductively-coupled plasma mass spectrometry (ICP-MS) (Agilent, Santa Clara, CA, USA) was performed for muscle sample metal ion analysis. Intramuscular metal ion concentration was determined using a four-point linear curve of analyte-standard response ratio.

Immunohistochemical staining of ZIP14 in human muscle sections

Human muscle tissue sections were obtained from autopsy cases from the University of Nebraska Medical Center (UNMC) with approval from the Institutional Review Board (IRB). In brief, formalin-fixed paraffin-embedded pectoralis and diaphragm muscles from non-cachectic and cachectic metastatic pancreatic adenocarcinoma patients were sectioned at 5μm-thickness onto positive-charged glass slides. Slides were incubated at 60°C for an hour and rehydrated using Histo-clear (National Diagnostics, Atlanta, GA, USA) and a series of ethanol gradients. Endogenous peroxide was blocked in 1% hydrogen peroxide for 10 min at room temperature. Antigen retrieval was performed using citrate buffer, pH 6.0 (Vector laboratories, Burlingame, CA, USA) in a steamer apparatus for 30 min. All remaining incubation steps were performed at room temperature with three PBS washes between each incubation step. Endogenous avidin and biotin were blocked using avidin and biotin blocking reagents (Vector laboratories, Burlingame, CA, USA), respectively for 15 min each. Tissues were then blocked with PBS containing 2% BSA and 10% goat serum for 30 min and then incubated with rabbit polyclonal antibody against human ZIP14 (developed in our laboratory as referenced[171]) at 1:1000 dilution within blocking buffer. Tissues were then incubated in biotinylated goat anti-rabbit IgG secondary antibody (Vector laboratories, Burlingame, CA, USA) at 1:250 dilution within blocking buffer. The ABC and DAB kits (Vector laboratories, Burlingame, CA, USA) were used for signal amplification and detection, respectively, according to manufacturer's instructions. Tissues were then counterstained with hematoxylin (Richard-Allan Scientific, Kalamazoo, MI, USA), dehydrated, and cover slides were mounted using Cytoseal XYL (Richard-Allan Scientific, Kalamazoo, MI, USA) for histological analysis. ZIP14-stained pectoralis and diaphragm muscles from non cachectic and cachectic adenocarcinoma patients were scored as ZIP14-positive or -negative in a blinded pathological analysis.

Muscle sample immunoblot analysis

15 mg of snap frozen gastrocnemius muscles from FC1242 and Pan02 experimental metastasis models and healthy control mice were homogenized in 250μL of lysis buffer containing 150mM NaCl, 0.5% sodium deoxycholate, 1% NP-40, and 0.1% SDS in 50mM Tris pH8.0 supplemented with protease inhibitor (Roche, Mannheim, Germany) and phosphate inhibitor (Thermo Scientific, Waltham, MA, USA). Muscle samples were lysed using the TissueLyser II (Qiagen, Hilden, Germany) for two three minute cycles and supernatants were isolated after centrifugation at 15,000 x g for 15 min. The BCA protein assay (Pierce, Thermo Fisher Scientific, Carlsbad, CA, USA) was performed on supernatants to determine protein concentration. Proteins were run on an SDS-PAGE gel, transferred onto a nitrocellulose membrane, and blocked for an hour with 5% non-fat milk in 25mmol/L Tris-HCl pH7.4 supplemented with 150mmol/L NaCl and 0.1% Tween20 (TBS-T). Membranes were incubated with rabbit antibody against ZIP14 (developed in our laboratory as referenced[171]) at 1:500 dilution, followed by goat anti-rabbit IgG secondary antibody and HRP-conjugated donkey anti-goat IgG tertiary antibody (Sigma, St. Louis, MO, USA). Membranes were also incubated with rabbit antibody against GAPDH (Cell Signaling

Technologies, Beverly, MA, USA) as a loading control, followed by HRP-conjugated goat anti-rabbit IgG secondary antibody (Sigma, St. Louis, MO, USA). Membranes were developed using the ECL substrate (Bio-rad, Hercules, CA, USA) and visualized using the Bio-Rad ChemiDoc Imaging System (Rio-Rad, Heracules, CA, USA).

Statistical Analysis

Statistical analysis for body weight, hind-limb grip strength, muscle fiber cross-sectional areas, and gene expression were performed using the unpaired, two-tailed Student's t-test using the GraphPad Prism 8 (GraphPad Software, San Diego, CA, USA) software. Statistical analysis for ZIP14-stained human pectoralis and diaphragm muscle sections was performed using the Pearson's chi-square test. All values are shown as the mean $\pm$ standard error of the mean (SEM). p-values of < 0.05 are considered to be statistically significant.

Human Specimens

Human patient pancreatic adenocarcinoma, metastatic lesions, pectoralis and diaphragm muscles, and unaffected samples from descendants previously diagnosed with pancreatic adenocarcinoma were obtained prospectively from the UNMC Tissue Bank through the Rapid Autopsy Program (RAP) for Pancreas. The RAP at the UNMC operates with IRB compliance and the approval code: UNMC IRB 091-01, which requires donor and next-of-kin consent for the collection and usage of patient samples in research. The UNMC RAP is not classified as Human Subjects Research and is exempt under 45 CFR 46.101(b)(4) from 45 CFR part 46 requirements. Clinical data for each donor were obtained from multiple sources, including OneChat and the UNMC Pathology autopsy report, which contains patient height, weight, and observable donor characteristics. All patient sample and clinicopathological data were deidentified prior to distribution and listed in Table S2.

Pancreas, duodenal, spleen, liver, and diaphragm samples from non cancer patients were obtained through collaboration with Live On Nebraska. All patient samples and data were deidentified prior to distribution to UNMC and were stored under the auspices of the RAP. Limited deidentified patient clinical information was provided and listed in Table S2.

All organs and tissues were harvested within 3 hours postmortem and either flash frozen or fixed in formalin immediately to ensure retention of specimen quality. 5µm-thick sections were cut from formalin-fixed paraffin-embedded tissue onto positive charged slides for distribution.

Table S2: Rapid Autopsy Program (RAP) de-identified human patient information

A

RAP #	Age	Sex	Survival Days	Stage at Diagnosis	Stage at endpoint collection	Cachexia (1) Presence of cachexia: 1 and absence: 0
105	89	F	26	IV	IV	0
107	83	F	269	IV	IV	1 (minimal)
108	78	M	762	IIA	IV	1
109	64	M	405	IV	IV	1
110	36	M	138	IV	IV	1
111	43	M	326	IV	IV	0
112	84	F	21	IV	IV	0
113	58	F	878	IV	IV	1
115	80	M	63	IV	IV	0
116	80	F	497	IV	IV	1
117	68	M	316	III	IV	1
118	72	M	38	IV	IV	0
119	85	F	183	IV	IV	1
120	69	M	507	III	IV	1
121	75	F	235	III	IV	0
123	74	M	90	IV	IV	0
124	53	F	421	IV	IV	1
125	49	F	27	IV	IV	1
126	60	F	353	III	IV	1

B

RAP Non-cancer controls

RAP NORS ID	Age	Sex	Height (cm)	Weight (kg)
1	59	M	194	93
3	58	F	164	99
13	61	M	170	89
21	53	M	180	110
23	39	M	172	121
24	48	F	165	66
25	36	F	156	70
28	57	F	155	66
32	48	M	163	67

Table S2A-B: Limited de-identified human patient information. **(A)** Rapid Autopsy Program (RAP) #105-126: cachectic and non-cachectic pancreatic adenocarcinoma patients. **(B)** RAP NORS #1, 3, 13, 21, 23, 24, 25, 28 and 32: non-cachectic, non-cancer patients.

Chapter 3

Cell lines

The *Bard1*-deficient murine mammary carcinoma cells were isolated and derived from a primary mammary tumor from a Bard1$^{flex1/flex1}$, Wap$^{cre/+}$ *Bard1* mammary epithelium-specific conditional knockout genetically engineered mouse model with a B6129SF1/J background.[208] The cells were procured from the Baer laboratory (Columbia University, New York, NY, USA). *Bard1*-deficient murine mammary carcinoma cells were cultured in DMEM supplemented with 10% fetal bovine serum (Sigma, St. Louis, MO, USA), 1% penicillin/streptomycin (Life Technologies, Carlsbad, CA, USA) and grown in a 37ºC humidified incubator with 5% CO_2.

Mouse studies

All mouse studies, experiments, and protocols were approved by The Columbia University Institutional Animal Care and Use Committee (IACUC) and are compliant with ethical guidelines and regulations from the Institute of Comparative Medicine (ICM) at Columbia University Irving Medical Center (CUIMC) with the IACUC-approved protocol: AAAR6450. All mice were housed in CUIMC's pathogen-free barrier facility and fed on Labdiet 5053 (standard diet). Female 8- to 9-week old B6129SF1/J background mice were purchased from Jackson laboratory (Bar Harbor, ME, USA). Mice were orthotopically injected with 5 x 10^5 *Bard1*-deficient murine mammary carcinoma cells into the left fourth mammary fat pad. Mouse body weight and tumor volume were measured weekly. Tumor length and width were measured using digital calipers and the tumor volumes were calculated using the formula: Volume (mm^3) = ($Width^2$) x (Length/2). Mouse body condition, as an indicator of cachexia development, was determined by routine observation of mice as described previously.[306]

Measurement of body weight and hind-limb grip strength

Measurements of body weight from healthy control mice and orthotopic *Bard1*-deficient metastatic TNBC models were performed weekly using a bench-top digital balance. All body weight measurements were normalized to the body weight on the day of tumor cell injection (day 0 post injection). Measurements of hind-limb grip strength were taken weekly using a grip strength meter (Columbus Instruments, Columbia, OH, USA). A minimum of five measurements were performed per mouse weekly and the mean values were calculated. The percent grip strength was normalized to the mean initial grip strength values (100%) on the day of tumor cell injection.

Tissue Collection

Gastrocnemius, tibialis anterior, diaphragm, and heart muscles were harvested and fixed in 4% paraformaldehyde for 24 hours at 4°C or snap frozen in liquid nitrogen at stored at -80°C for histological analysis and molecular analysis, respectively. Liver and lung tissues were harvested and fixed in 4% paraformaldehyde for 24 hours at 4°C. All paraformaldehyde-fixed tissues were washed in PBS for an hour and stored in 70% ethanol until further histological processing and analysis.

Histological analysis of metastases and muscle fibers

For histological analysis, paraformaldehyde-fixed paraffin-embedded gastrocnemius and lung tissues were sectioned at 5μm-thickness onto positive-charged slides and stained with hematoxylin and eosin (H&E). H&E-stained gastrocnemius and diaphragm tissue sections were visualized and imaged using an Eclipse Ni-U microscope (Nikon Corporation, Tokyo, Japan). H&E-stained liver and lung tissue sections were visualized and imaged under a DM5500B microscope (Leica Microsystems, Wetzlar, Germany).

Analysis of muscle cross-sectional area

Random two or three fields, totaling a combined average of 250 individual muscle fibers, per H&E-stained paraformaldehyde-fixed paraffin-embedded 5μm-thick cross-sections of gastrocnemius muscles were imaged at 20x magnification using a DM5500B microscope (Leica Microsystems, Wetzlar, Germany). Muscle fiber cross-sectional area was quantified using the drawing module in ImageJ (ImageJ software, Version 1.52h, National Institutes of Health, Bethesda, MD, USA) to trace individual muscle fiber boundaries. Muscle fiber cross-sectional areas from tumor-bearing and control mice were stratified by cross-sectional area ranges of various sizes and the percentage of fibers in each range were calculated. The means of cross-sectional areas for each range were determined from replicate muscle samples.

RT-qPCR analysis of gene expression

Snap frozen gastrocnemius, tibialis anterior, diaphragm, and heart muscles were minced into ~1-2mm pieces and 15mg, representative of each sample, were taken from each muscle for total RNA extraction using Trizol (Life Technologies, Carlsbad, CA, USA). Muscle samples were lysed using 5mm steel beads (Qiagen, Hilden, Germany) and the TissueLyser II (Qiagen, Hilden, Germany) instrument. Samples were centrifuged at 18,000 x g for 5 min and the supernatant was isolated and processed using the RNeasy Mini Kit (Qiagen, Hilden, Germany) with DNase treatment while in-column, accounting to manufacturer's instructions. The total purified RNA in each sample was quantified using a Nanodrop spectrophotometer (Thermo Fisher Scientific, Walthom, MA, USA) and 500ng of RNA was reverse transcribed into cDNA using the cDNA Synthesis Kit (Applied Biosystems, Thermo Fisher Scientific, Walthom, MA, USA). RT-qPCR was performed using 10ng of cDNA from each sample mixed with gene-specific ptimers and SYBR Green PCR master mix (Applied Biosystems, Thermo Fisher Scientific, Walthom, MA, USA). Primers for *Gapdh* were used as an internal control. RT-qPCR data were analyzed on an Applied Biosystems 7500 Real Time PCR system (Applied Biosystems, Thermo Fisher Scientific, Walthom, MA, USA) and the fold change in gene expression was determined using the $2^{-\Delta\Delta DCt}$ method.[307] RT-qPCR primer sequences used in this study are shown in Table S1.

Intramuscular metal ion analysis

15-20mg of each gastrocnemius and diaphragm muscle were sent to the Veterinary Diagnostic Laboratory at Michigan State University, MI, USA, for metal ion analysis. Tissues were dried overnight at 75ºC, digested overnight in 10x volume relative to muscle dry weight of nitric acid, and diluted in a 100-fold volume of water. Inductively-coupled plasma mass spectrometry (ICP-MS) (Agilent, Santa Clara, CA, USA) was performed for muscle sample metal ion analysis. Intramuscular metal ion concentration was determined using a four-point linear curve of analyte-standard response ratio.

Muscle sample immunoblot analysis

15 mg of snap frozen gastrocnemius muscles from FC1242 and Pan02 experimental metastasis models and healthy control mice were homogenized in 250μL of lysis buffer containing 150mM NaCl, 0.5% sodium deoxycholate, 1% NP-40, and 0.1% SDS in 50mM Tris pH8.0 supplemented with protease inhibitor (Roche, Mannheim, Germany) and phosphate inhibitor (Thermo Scientific, Waltham, MA, USA). Muscle samples were lysed using the TissueLyser II (Qiagen, Hilden, Germany) for two three minute cycles and supernatants were isolated after centrifugation at 15,000 x g for 15 min. The BCA protein assay (Pierce, Thermo Fisher Scientific, Carlsbad, CA, USA) was performed on supernatants to determine protein concentration. Proteins were run on an SDS-PAGE gel, transferred onto nitrocellulose membrane, and blocked for an hour with 5% non-fat milk in 25mmol/L Tris-HCl pH7.4 supplemented with 150mmol/L NaCl and 0.1% Tween20 (TBS-T). Membranes were incubated with rabbit antibody against Phospho-SMAD2 and SMAD2 (Cell Signaling Technologies, Beverly, MA, USA) at 1:500 dilution, followed by incubation with goat anti-rabbit IgG secondary antibody and HRP-conjugated donkey anti-goat IgG tertiary antibody (Sigma, St. Louis, MO, USA). Membranes were also incubated with mouse antibody against skeletal actin (Sigma, St Louis, MO, USA) at 1:5000 dilution as an internal control, followed by HRP-conjugated anti-mouse IgG secondary antibody (Sigma, St. Louis, MO, USA). Membranes were developed using the ECL substrate (Bio-rad, Hercules, CA, USA) and visualized using the Bio-Rad ChemiDoc Imaging System (Rio-Rad, Heracules, CA, USA).

Chapter 4

Cell lines

The 4T1 murine triple-negative breast cancer cell line was derived from the 410.4 cell line, which was isolated from a primary mammary tumor that developed spontaneously from a MMTV$^+$ mouse with a BALB/c background.[232,308] The 4T1 cell line was kindly provided by the Kang laboratory (Princeton University, Princeton, NJ, USA). The LM3 murine triple-negative breast cancer cell line was derived from the M3 cell line, which was isolated from a primary mammary tumor that developed spontaneously from a BALB/c background mouse.[234] The LM3 cell line was kindly provided by the Urtreger laboratory (University of Buenos Aires, Buenos Aires, Argentina). The 4T1 and LM3 cells were cultured in RPMI-1640 and MEM, respectively, supplemented with 10% fetal bovine serum (Sigma, St. Louis, MO, USA) and 1% penicillin/streptomycin (Life Technologies, Carlsbad, CA, USA). Cell lines were grown in a 37°C humidified incubator with 5% CO_2.

Mouse studies

All mouse studies, experiments, and protocols were approved by The Columbia University Institutional Animal Care and Use Committee (IACUC) and are compliant with ethical guidelines and regulations from the Institute of Comparative Medicine (ICM) at Columbia University Irving Medical Center (CUIMC) with the IACUC-approved protocol: AABF2565. All mice were housed in CUIMC's pathogen-free barrier facility and fed on Labdiet 5053 (standard diet). Female, 6- to 8-week old BALB/cJ (Stock No: 000651) and B cell-deficient Igh-J^{tm1Cgn} (Jh) mice (Model # 1147-F) with a BALB/c background were purchased from Jackson laboratories (Bar Harbor, ME, USA) and Taconic Biosciences (Rensselaer, NY, USA), respectively. 4T1 and LM3 orthotopic metastasis models were generated by orthotopic injection of 5×10^5 4T1 cells or 1×10^6 LM3 cells into the left fourth mammary fat pad of syngeneic BALB/cJ or BALB/c background mice. 4T1 and LM3 experimental metastasis models were generated by intravenous injection 1×10^5 tumor cells into the tail vein of syngeneic BALB/cJ mice. Primary tumor growth was measured semi-weekly by digital calipers. 4T1 orthotopic metastasis models were euthanized at either 15 days or 3 weeks post tumor cell-implantation for early and late metastasis timepoints, respectively. LM3 orthotopic metastasis models were euthanized at 4 weeks post tumor cell-implantation. 4T1 and LM3 experimental metastasis models were euthanized at 3 weeks post tumor cell-injection.

Human Specimens

The Molecular Pathology Shared Resource (MPSR) Tissue Bank at the New York Presbyterian Hospital/Columbia University Irving Medical Center operates in compliance HIPAA guidelines and institutional review board (IRB)-approved protocols, and is licensed by the New York State Department of Health. 5μm-thick, formalin-fixed, paraffin-embedded metastatic lung sections from human triple-negative breast cancer patients were obtained from the MPSR Tissue Bank in compliance with the IRB-approved protocol: IRB-AAAR1682. The presence of triple-negative breast cancer and lung metastasis from each patient sample was confirmed by two independent pathologists at the Columbia University Irving Medical Center. Limited deidentified patient clinical information was provided and listed in Table S3.

Table S3: Molecular Pathology Shared Resource (MPSR) Tissue Bank de-identified human triple-negative breast cancer patient information

Triple-negative breast cancer patient number	Tumor-infiltrating B cell density score
SP18-9267	Low
SP97-13426	Low
SP04-5220	High

SP14-2468	High
SP17-4319	High
SP06-21017	High
SP16-17328	Low
SP14-12956	Low
SP19-6496	High
SP04-11676	Low
SP09-3187	Low
SP09-14522	Low
SP11-25325	High
SP13-13241	High
SP13-27453	High

Table S3: Limited de-identified human triple-negative breast cancer patient information. Molecular Pathology Shared Resource (MPSR) Tissue Bank # SP18-9267, SP97-13426, SP04-5220, SP14-2468, SP17-4319, SP06-21017, SP16-17328, SP14-12956, SP19-6496, SP04-11676, SP09-3187, SP09-14522, SP11-25325, SP13-13241, SP13-27453: triple-negative breast cancer patients. Tumor-infiltrating B cell density for each patient sample was determined independently by a pathologist as low (0, +, and ++) or high (+++ and ++++).

Tissue Collection

Primary tumors and metastatic lungs were harvested and fixed in 4% paraformaldehyde for 24 hours at 4°C, washed in PBS for an hour, and stored in 70% ethanol until further histological processing and analysis.

Histological analysis of metastases and muscle fibers

For histological analysis, paraformaldehyde-fixed lung tissues were embedded in paraffin blocks and sectioned at 5μm-thickness onto positive-charged slides and stained with hematoxylin and eosin (H&E). The presence of lung metastases was determined through visualization of H&E-stained lung sections using an Eclipse Ni-U microscope (Nikon Corporation, Tokyo, Japan).

Immunohistochemical staining

Paraformaldehyde-fixed, paraffin-embedded lungs from tumor-bearing mice were sectioned at 5μm-thickness onto positively charged glass slides. Formalin-fixed, paraffin-embedded metastatic lung sections from human triple-negative breast cancer patients were obtained from the Molecular Pathology Shared Resource (MPSR) Tissue Bank at the New York Presbyterian/Columbia University Irving Medical Center with the institutional review board (IRB)-approved protocol: IRB-AAAR1682. Slides were incubated at 60°C for an hour and rehydrated using Histo-clear (National Diagnostics, Atlanta, GA, USA) and a series of ethanol gradients. Endogenous peroxide was blocked in 1% hydrogen peroxide for 10 min at room temperature. Antigen retrieval was performed using citrate buffer, pH 6.0 (Vector laboratories, Burlingame, CA, USA) or Tris-alkaline buffer, pH8.0 (Vector laboratories, Burlingame, CA, USA) a steamer apparatus for 30 min. All remaining incubation steps were performed at room temperature with three PBS washes between each incubation step. Endogenous avidin and biotin were blocked using avidin and biotin blocking reagents (Vector laboratories, Burlingame, CA, USA), respectively for 15 min each. Tissues were then blocked with PBS containing 3% BSA and 10% goat or rabbit serum for 30 min and then incubated with primary antibodies (Table S4). For chromogenic staining, tissues were then incubated in biotinylated secondary antibodies (Table S4) at 1:250 dilution within blocking buffer for 30 min. The ABC and DAB kits (Vector laboratories, Burlingame, CA, USA) were used for signal amplification and detection, respectively, according to manufacturer's instructions. Tissues were then counterstained with hematoxylin (Richard-Allan Scientific, Kalamazoo, MI, USA), dehydrated, and cover slides were mounted using Cytoseal XYL (Richard-Allan Scientific, Kalamazoo, MI, USA) for histological analysis. For immunofluorescent staining, slides were incubated in fluorophore-conjugated secondary antibodies (Table S4) for 30 min in the dark. Tissue autofluorescence was quenched using the Vector TrueVIEW

Autofluorescence Quenching Kit (Vector Laboratories, Buringame, CA, USA) according to manufacturer's instructions. Slides were mounted using Fluoro-Gel II with DAPI (Electron Microscopy Sciences, Hatfield, PA, USA).

Table S4: Primary and secondary antibodies utilized for immunohistochemical and immunofluorescent staining

Antibody	Catalogue Number	Manufacturer	Concentration
Rat anti-mouse B220 Biotin Conjugated	BD553085	BD Biosciences, CA	1:200
Rabbit anti-mouse S100A9	73425S	Cell Signaling, MA	1:2000
Rabbit anti-mouse PAX-5	12709S	Cell Signaling, MA	1:100
Mouse anti-human CD20	MS340-S	ThermoMab, CA	1:100
Rabbit anti-mouse / human Keratin-14	905301	Biolegend, CA	1:5,000
Rabbit anti-mouse / human phospho-mTOR (Ser2448)	2976S	Cell Signaling, MA	1:400
Goat Anti-Rabbit IgG (H+L) Biotinylated	BA-1000	Vector Labs, CA	1:250
Rabbit Anti-Rat IgG (H+L) Biotinylated	BA-4001	Vector Labs, CA	1:250
Goat anti-Rabbit IgG (H+L) Cross-Adsorbed Secondary Antibody, Alexa Fluor 568	A-11011	ThermoFisher Scientific, MA	1:250
Goat anti-Rat IgG (H+L) Cross-Adsorbed Secondary Antibody, Alexa Fluor 488	A-11006	ThermoFisher Scientific, MA	1:250

Table S4: Information for primary and secondary antibodies used for immunohistochemical and immunofluorescent staining

Analysis of immunohistochemistry-stained tissues

Chromogen-stained metastatic lung sections were visualized and imaged using an Eclipse Ni-U microscope (Nikon Corporation, Tokyo, Japan). The number of positive-stained cells and the number and surface area of each lung metastasis were quantified using the counting and drawing modules of the ImageJ software (Version 1.53c, National Institute of Health, Bethesda, MD, USA), respectively. The spatial localization of metastasis-infiltrating, positive-stained B cells in mouse tissue were classified as invasive margin or interior based on the following criteria: invasive margin: within a 10μm, or 20μm, or 30μm margin from the edge of the metastasis toward the interior for areas with a width of under 50μm, 51-100μm, or over 100μm; interior: outside of the defined invasive margin toward the interior of the metastasis. The spatial localization of metastasis-infiltrating positive-stained B cells in human triple-negative breast cancer patient lung sections were classified as invasive margin or interior localization as described[309] using the region-of-interest drawing and positive cell detection modules of the Quantitative Pathology & Bioimage Analysis software (QuPath Version 2.0, University of Edinburgh, Edinburgh, United Kingdom). Only lung sections showing complete lung metastases, defined as without artefacts in the interior and the invasive margin and without with sections of the lung metastases cut off, from human triple-negative breast cancer patients were analyzed. Metastasis-infiltrating B cells located further within the metastasis from the defined invasive margin region are classified as interior localization. B cell counts were calculated as 1) the proportion of the number of invasive margin or interior localization B cells to total B cells (with all counts normalized to the surface area of each lung metastasis, and 2) the ratio of total metastasis-infiltrating B cells to the number of tumor cells in each lung metastasis. Cytoekratin-14- and p-mTOR-stained lung metastases from mouse models were analyzed as the proportion of positive-stained tumor cells to total tumor cells in each metastasis using the region-of-interest drawing and positive cell detection module of the Quantitative Pathology & Bioimage Analysis software (QuPath Version 2.0, University of Edinburgh, Edinburgh, United Kingdom). Tumor cells were identified by restricting the cell detection parameters to large-nucleated cells and positive staining was detected by setting thresholds for signal intensity (low: 1+, high: 2+ and 3+). The number of lung metastases for 4T1 orthotopic metastasis models harvested at 15 days post tumor cell-injection was calculated by the quantitation of the number metastases and the number of tumor cells in each metastasis from 5 cytokeratin-14-stained lung sections taken at $\geq$20µm intervals for each mouse. Representative images were taken at 20x magnification using an Eclipse Ni-U microscope (Nikon Corporation, Tokyo, Japan). CD20-stained metastatic lungs from human triple-negative breast cancer patients were scored as having low (0, +, and ++) or high (+++ and ++++) numbers of tumor-infiltrating B cells in a blinded pathological review by an independent pathologist. p-mTOR-stained lung metastases from human triple-negative breast cancer patients were scored as low (0 and +) or high (++ and +++) expression in a blinded pathological review. Immunofluorescent-stained metastatic lungs were visualized and imaged using a Leica CTR5500 microscope with a Leica DFC3000 G camera module (Leica Microsystems, Wetzlar, Germany). Positive cells were determined using the counting module of the ImageJ software (Version 1.53c, National Institute of Health, Bethesda, MD, USA). All data is representative of a minimum of 3 independent experiments.

Isolation of lung metastases and development of lung-metastasis-derived organoids

Lungs with macroscopic metastatic lesions from 4T1 and LM3 orthotopic metastasis models were harvested, briefly washed in ice-cold HBSS, and minced with a scalpel into 1-2mm^3 pieces.[310,311] Minced tissues were transferred into a 15mL tube and digested in 0.1% Collagenase I (Worthington Biochemical, Lakewood, NJ, USA), 0.1% Trypsin (Sigma, St. Louis, MO, USA), 0.1% Insulin (Sigma, St. Louis, MO, USA), and 1% Penicillin/Streptomycin (Life Technologies, Carlsbad, CA, USA) in DMEM High Glucose medium for 30-45 min at 37°C on a shaker until broken into barely-visible pieces and not over-digested.[310] Digested tissues were pelleted by centrifugation at 1500 rpm for 10 min and the supernatant was removed. The organoid pellet was resuspended and washed in DMEM, then centrifuged at 1,500 rpm for 10 min and the supernatant was aspirated. The organoid pellet was resuspended in 4mL DMEM containing 40µL of 2000 U/mL DNase (Sigma, St. Louis, MO, USA) and mixed for 5 min by gentle inversion of the tube by hand. The organoids were then subjected to 5 spin-wash cycles with DMEM. After the final cycle, the organoid pellet was re-suspended in 1-2mL DMEM.

Organoid plating and passaging

Organoid density was calculated and re-adjusted to the desired concentration of 1000 organoids per mL of solution.[310] Briefly, a 40µL sample of resuspended organoids was pipetted onto a 30mm petri dish to determine the concentration of organoids in the solution.[312] The volume of organoid solution needed to acquired the desired number of organoids was calculated and aliquoted into a 1.5mL microcentrifuge tube and pelleted by centrifugation at 300 x g. The supernatant was aspirated and resuspended in the desired amount of Matrigel (pre-thawed overnight in 4°C and kept on ice until use) according to the following formula calculated for plating onto a 12-well plate: aliquot volume = number of wells × 50 organoids / concentration of organoid solution. 40µL of the Matrigel-suspended organoids were then plated onto each well of a 12-well plate. The plated organoids were incubated at 37°C for 30 min for the Matrigel to fully solidify and 1.5mL of medium respective of the organoid cell line (DMEM or RPMI-1640 supplemented with 10% Fetal Bovine Serum (Sigma, St. Louis, MO, USA) and 1% penicillin/streptomycin (Life Technologies, Carlsbad, CA, USA)) was added into each well. Organoid cultures were passaged weekly by aspirating the medium and dissociation of the Matrigel matrix by adding 1mL of ice-cold PBS. Organoids were mechanically dissociated into smaller pieces by pipetting up and down using a P1000 pipette. Once the Matrigel and organoids was dissolved and broken down, respectively, the organoid suspension was transferred into a 1.5mL microcentrifuge tube and spun down at 300 x g for 5 min at 4°C. The supernatant was removed from the tube using a P200 pipette. Organoids were resuspended in fresh Matrigel (volume of Matrigel added = number of wells x 40 µL) plating onto a 12-well plate: aliquot volume = number of wells × 50 organoids / concentration of organoid solution. 40µL of the Matrigel-suspended organoids were then plated onto each well of a 12-well plate. The plated organoids were incubated at 37°C for 30 min for the Matrigel to fully solidify and 1.5mL of medium respective of the organoid cell line (DMEM or RPMI-1640 supplemented with 10% Fetal Bovine Serum and 1% penicillin/streptomycin (Life Technologies, Carlsbad, CA, USA)) was added into each well.

Isolation of B cells by flow cytometry

4T1 and LM3 orthotopic metastasis models were euthanized and their lungs and blood were extracted according to Columbia University's Institutional Animal Care and Use Committee's approved protocol: AABF2565. Lungs were washed in ice-cold sterile HBSS and transferred into a sterile hood. Lungs were minced with a scalpel into 1-2mm^3 pieces followed by transfer into a 15mL tube and digested in digestion buffer, HBSS supplemented with 2mg/mL collagenase I (Worthington Biochemical, Lakewood, NJ, USA), and 2 U/mL dispase II (Roche, Indianapolis, IN, USA), and incubated at 37°C for 30 min on a shaker. Digested lung tissues were pelleted by centrifugation at 500 x g for 5 min at 4°C. The supernatant was aspirated and the pellet was resuspended in sterile HBSS at 4°C. Blood was collected by cardiac puncture and immediately transferred into BD Vacutainer plastic blood collection tubes with K_2EDTA (BD Biosciences, San Jose, CA, USA). Red blood cells were lysed with 2-3mL/lung or 1mL/100µL blood of ACK Lysis Buffer (Lonza, Morristown, NJ, USA) for 3 minutes and quenched by adding 8mL of sterile HBSS at 4°C. Cells were passed through a 70µm filter, centrifuged at 500 x g for 5 min, resuspended in

sterile HBSS, centrifuged again, and resuspended in FACS buffer (HBSS + 0.5% BSA) at 4°C.
Cell concentration was calculated using a TC20 Automated Cell Counter (Bio-Rad, Hercules, CA,
USA). The desired cell concentration was adjusted and transferred into 1.5mL microcentrifuge
tubes and stained with fluorophore conjugated antibodies at 1:100 (Table S5) for 45 min at 4°C. B
cells were sorted using the BD Influx cell sorter (BD Biosciences, San Jose, CA, USA). Sorted B
cells were pelleted at 500 x g, the supernatant was aspirated, and resuspended in B cell medium:
RPMI-1640 supplemented with 10% Fetal Bovine Serum (Sigma, St. Louis, MO, USA), 2mM L-
glutamine (Sigma, St. Louis, MO, USA), and 0.5µM 2-mercaptoethanol (Sigma, St. Louis, MO,
USA). B cells were plated onto sterile 30mm petri dishes and incubated overnight in a 37°C
humidified incubator with 5% CO_2.

Table S5: Antibodies utilized for flow cytometry experiments

Antibody	Fluorochrome Conjugate	Catalogue Number	Manufacturer
Rat IgG2b κ anti-mouse CD45	PerCP	BD557235	BD Biosciences, CA
Rat IgG2a κ anti-mouse B220	FITC	BD553087	BD Biosciences, CA
Rat IgG2a κ Isotype Control	PE	12-4321-71	eBiosciences, CA
Rat IgG2b κ isotype Control	PE	BD553989	BD Biosciences, CA

Table S4: Information for antibodies used for flow cytometry experiments

3-Dimensional co-culture of lung metastases-derived organoids and sorted B cells

Organoids were passaged and resuspended in ice-cold Matrigel as previously described
(volume of Matrigel added = number of wells x 40 µL). Sorted B cells were cultured overnight

133

and the concentration was determined using a TC20 Automated Cell Counter (Bio-Rad, Hercules, CA, USA). The volume needed to acquire the desired number of B cells was determined using the formula: 1×10^4 B cells / well (12-well plate), and aliquoted into a 1.5mL microcentrifuge tube. The B cells were spun at 1,500 rpm and the supernatant was aspirated. The organoid-Matrigel mixture was then transferred into the B cell tube and both organoids and B cells were homogeneously resuspended through gentle pipetting on ice. 40μL of organoid and B cell suspension in Matrigel was added on each well of a 12-well plate. The plated organoids were incubated at 37°C for 30 min for the Matrigel to fully solidify and 1.5mL of medium respective of the organoid cell line (DMEM or RPMI-1640 supplemented with 10% Fetal Bovine Serum (Sigma, St. Louis, MO, USA) and 1% penicillin/streptomycin (Life Technologies, Carlsbad, CA, USA) was added into each well. Organoids were imaged at 10x magnification at 0, 48, and 96 hours post plating using a Leica DM IL LED microscope (Leica Microsystems, Wetzlar, Germany). [312]. Data is representative of a minimum of three independent experiments. Data is representative of a minimum of three independent experiments.

Quantitation of 3-dimensional organoid invasion

Monoculture control and co-cultured lung metastasis-derived organoids were imaged at 10x magnification at 0, 48, and 96 hours post plating using a Leica DM IL LED microscope (Leica Microsystems, Wetzlar, Germany). Organoid invasion was calculated by outlining and calculating the form factor of each organoid using the drawing module and shape descriptors plugin of ImageJ (ImageJ software, Version 1.52h, National Institutes of Health, Bethesda, MD, USA). The form factor formula is as follows: Form Factor = (Perimeter)^2 / (4πArea). A perfect circle has a form factor of 1, which is the maximum area for a given perimeter, and organoids with increasing irregular shapes and invasive protrusions will have increased form factors. Invasion over time is quantified as a measure of fold change of form factor over time.

Transwell migration assay

For each well used for the transwell migration assay: 5×10^4 tumor cells were serum-starved overnight in serum-low medium, RPMI-1640 supplemented with 0.2% Fetal Bovine Serum (Sigma, St. Louis, MO, USA) and 1% penicillin/streptomycin (Life Technologies, Carlsbad, CA, USA), with or without 1×10^4 B220$^+$ B cells isolated from the lungs of orthotopic metastasis models and suspended in a Millicell PET 0.4µm-pore size membrane hanging cell culture insert (Millipore, Burlington, MA, USA) containing B cell medium, RPMI-1640 supplemented with 10% Fetal Bovine Serum (Sigma, St. Louis, MO, USA), 2mM L-glutamine (Sigma, St. Louis, MO, USA), and 0.5µM 2-mercaptoethanol (Sigma, St. Louis, MO, USA). After overnight co-culture, B cells were removed and tumor cells were labeled with 5µM Celltracker Green CMFDA dye (Life Technologies, Carlsbad, CA, USA) for 30 min. Tumors cells were trypsinized and resuspended in a 24 well-sized Corning Fluoroblok 3.0µm-pore size membrane cell culture insert (Corning Incorporated, Corning, NY, USA) containing serum-low medium, RPMI-1640 supplemented with 0.2% Fetal Bovine Serum (Sigma, St. Louis, MO, USA) and 1% penicillin/streptomycin (Life Technologies, Carlsbad, CA, USA). The inserts were placed into wells of a 24 well plate containing growth medium, RPMI-1640 supplemented with 10% Fetal Bovine Serum (Sigma, St. Louis, MO, USA), 1% penicillin/streptomycin (Life Technologies, Carlsbad, CA, USA) and incubated for 5 hours at 37°C in a humidified incubator with 5% CO_2 for tumor cell migration. After 5 hours, all media in the transwell and 24 well plate were aspirated. The transwells were washed in PBS and fixed in 4% paraformaldehyde for 15 min and washed twice with PBS. The cells on the apical side of each transwell membrane were gently scraped off and the membranes were excised using a scapel and forceps and mounted basal side up onto slides using Fluoro-Gel II with DAPI (Electron Microscopy Sciences, Hatfield, PA, USA). The total number of tumor cells that had fully migrated to the basal side of each transwell membrane were visualized and imaged at 10x magnification using a Leica CTR5500 microscope with a Leica DFC3000 G camera module (Leica Microsystems, Wetzlar, Germany) using the Leica Application Suite X software (Version 1.5.1.13187, Leica Microsystems, Wetzlar, Germany). The total number of tumor cells that had fully migrated to the basal side of each transwell membrane were counted using the counting module of ImageJ (ImageJ software, Version 1.52h, National Institutes of Health, Bethesda, MD, USA). Tumor cells located on the outer edges of the membrane were excluded from all counts to exclude artifactual edge-effects. Data is representative of a minimum of three independent experiments.

p-mTOR immunoblot analysis

5×10^4 tumor cells were cultured in growth medium, RPMI-1640 supplemented with 10% Fetal Bovine Serum (Sigma, St. Louis, MO, USA), 1% penicillin/streptomycin (Life Technologies, Carlsbad, CA, USA), with or without 1×10^4 B220$^+$ B cells isolated from the lungs of orthotopic metastasis models and suspended in a Millicell PET 0.4μm-pore size membrane hanging cell culture insert (Millipore, Burlington, MA, USA) containing B cell medium, RPMI-1640 supplemented with 10% Fetal Bovine Serum (Sigma, St. Louis, MO, USA), 2mM L-glutamine (Sigma, St. Louis, MO, USA), and 0.5μM 2-mercaptoethanol (Sigma, St. Louis, MO, USA). After overnight co-culture, B cells were removed and tumor cells were lysed in lysis buffer containing 150mM NaCl, 0.5% sodium deoxycholate, 1% NP-40, and 0.1% SDS in 50mM Tris pH8.0 supplemented with protease inhibitor (Roche, Mannheim, Germany) and phosphate inhibitor (Thermo Scientific, Waltham, MA, USA). The BCA protein assay (Pierce, Thermo Fisher

Scientific, Carlsbad, CA, USA) was performed on supernatants to determine protein concentration. Proteins were run on an SDS-PAGE gel, transferred onto nitrocellulose membrane, and blocked for an hour with 5% non-fat milk in 25mmol/L Tris-HCl pH7.4 supplemented with 150mmol/L NaCl and 0.1% Tween20 (TBS-T). Membranes were incubated with rabbit antibody against mouse phosphor-mTOR at Ser2448 (Cell Signaling Technologies, Beverly, MA, USA) at 1:500 dilution, followed by incubation with goat anti-rabbit IgG secondary antibody and HRP-conjugated donkey anti-goat IgG tertiary antibody (Sigma, St. Louis, MO, USA). Membranes were also incubated with mouse antibody against skeletal actin (Sigma, St Louis, MO, USA) at 1:5000 dilution as an internal control, followed by HRP-conjugated anti-mouse secondary antibody (Sigma, St. Louis, MO, USA). Membranes were developed using the ECL substrate (Bio-rad, Hercules, CA, USA) and visualized using the Bio-Rad ChemiDoc Imaging System (Rio-Rad, Heracules, CA, USA).

Statistical analysis

Statistical significance for comparison of organoid invasion and fold change in form factor was calculated using the non-parametric unpaired Mann-Whitney U test, as these data do not follow a normal distribution. All other statistical significance between groups were determined using the unpaired two-tailed Student's *t*-test. All statistical analyses were calculated using the Prism Software (Version 9.1.0, GraphPad Software, San Diego, CA). Values are shown as either bar graphs (mean $\pm$ standard error of the mean) or as a violin plot (median, with the violin depicting the maximum and minimum of the dataset, respectively). A p-value of <0.05 was considered statistically significant. The specific test used for each experiment are listed in each figure legend.

References

1. Hajdu, S.I. A note from history: Landmarks in history of cancer, part 1. *Cancer* **117**, 1097-1102 (2011).

2. Society, A.C. Cancer Facts & Figures 2021. *American Cancer Society* (2021).

3. Siegel, R.L., Miller, K.D., Fuchs, H.E. & Jemal, A. Cancer Statistics, 2021. *CA: A Cancer Journal for Clinicians* **71**, 7-33 (2021).

4. Lambert, A.W., Pattabiraman, D.R. & Weinberg, R.A. Emerging Biological Principles of Metastasis. *Cell* **168**, 670-691 (2017).

5. Telloni, S.M. Tumor Staging and Grading: A Primer. in *Molecular Profiling: Methods and Protocols* (ed. Espina, V.) 1-17 (Springer New York, New York, NY, 2017).

6. Bross, I.D.J., Viadana, E. & Pickren, J.W. The metastatic spread of myeloma and leukemias in men. *Virchows Archiv A* **365**, 91-101 (1975).

7. Androutsos, G., *et al.* Joseph-Claude-Anthelme Récamier (1774-1852): forerunner in surgical oncology. *J buon* **16**, 572-576 (2011).

8. Virchow, R. Cellular pathology. As based upon physiological and pathological histology. Lecture XVI--Atheromatous affection of arteries. 1858. *Nutr Rev* **47**, 23-25 (1989).

9. Paget, S. THE DISTRIBUTION OF SECONDARY GROWTHS IN CANCER OF THE BREAST. *The Lancet* **133**, 571-573 (1889).

10. Fidler, I.J. The pathogenesis of cancer metastasis: the 'seed and soil' hypothesis revisited. *Nature Reviews Cancer* **3**, 453-458 (2003).

11. Akhtar, M., Haider, A., Rashid, S. & Al-Nabet, A.D.M.H. Paget's "Seed and Soil" Theory of Cancer Metastasis: An Idea Whose Time has Come. *Advances in Anatomic Pathology* **26**, 69-74 (2019).

12. Lucké, B., Breedis, C., Woo, Z.P., Berwick, L. & Nowell, P. Differential Growth of Metastatic Tumors in Liver and Lung. *Cancer Res* **12**, 734 (1952).

13. Sugarbaker, E.V. Cancer metastasis: A product of tumor-host interactions. *Current Problems in Cancer* **3**, 1-59 (1979).

14. Hart, I.R. & Fidler, I.J. Role of Organ Selectivity in the Determination of Metastatic Patterns of B16 Melanoma. *Cancer Res* **40**, 2281 (1980).

15. Morikawa, K., Walker, S.M., Jessup, J.M. & Fidler, I.J. In vivo selection of highly metastatic cells from surgical specimens of different primary human colon carcinomas implanted into nude mice. *Cancer Res* **48**, 1943-1948 (1988).

16.   Fidler, I.J. Selection of successive tumour lines for metastasis. *Nat New Biol* **242**, 148-149 (1973).

17.   Fidler, I.J. Metastasis: Quantitative Analysis of Distribution and Fate of Tumor Emboli Labeled With 125I-5-Iodo-2' -deoxyuridine23. *JNCI: Journal of the National Cancer Institute* **45**, 773-782 (1970).

18.   Gupta, G.P. & Massagué, J. Cancer Metastasis: Building a Framework. *Cell* **127**, 679-695 (2006).

19.   Thiery, J.P. Epithelial–mesenchymal transitions in tumour progression. *Nature Reviews Cancer* **2**, 442-454 (2002).

20.   Bernards, R. & Weinberg, R.A. Metastasis genes: A progression puzzle. *Nature* **418**, 823-823 (2002).

21.   Yu, M., *et al.* Circulating breast tumor cells exhibit dynamic changes in epithelial and mesenchymal composition. *Science (New York, N.Y.)* **339**, 580-584 (2013).

22.   Luzzi, K.J., *et al.* Multistep nature of metastatic inefficiency: dormancy of solitary cells after successful extravasation and limited survival of early micrometastases. *The American journal of pathology* **153**, 865-873 (1998).

23.   Chen, M.-T., *et al.* Comparison of patterns and prognosis among distant metastatic breast cancer patients by age groups: a SEER population-based analysis. *Scientific Reports* **7**, 9254 (2017).

24.   Vilalta, M., Rafat, M. & Graves, E.E. Effects of radiation on metastasis and tumor cell migration. *Cell Mol Life Sci* **73**, 2999-3007 (2016).

25.   Gianfaldoni, S., *et al.* An Overview on Radiotherapy: From Its History to Its Current Applications in Dermatology. *Open Access Maced J Med Sci* **5**, 521-525 (2017).

26.   Grubbé, E.H. Priority in the Therapeutic Use of X-rays. *Radiology* **21**, 156-162 (1933).

27.   Rossari, F., Zucchinetti, C., Buda, G. & Orciuolo, E. Tumor dormancy as an alternative step in the development of chemoresistance and metastasis - clinical implications. *Cellular Oncology* **43**, 155-176 (2020).

28.   Mansoori, B., Mohammadi, A., Davudian, S., Shirjang, S. & Baradaran, B. The Different Mechanisms of Cancer Drug Resistance: A Brief Review. *Adv Pharm Bull* **7**, 339-348 (2017).

29.   Rivera, E. & Gomez, H. Chemotherapy resistance in metastatic breast cancer: the evolving role of ixabepilone. *Breast Cancer Research* **12**, S2 (2010).

30.   Wong, S.T. & Goodin, S. Overcoming Drug Resistance in Patients with Metastatic Breast Cancer. *Pharmacotherapy: The Journal of Human Pharmacology and Drug Therapy* **29**, 954-965 (2009).

31.   Liu, Z., *et al.* Predicting distant metastasis and chemotherapy benefit in locally advanced rectal cancer. *Nat Commun* **11**, 4308 (2020).

32.   Januchowski, R., Wojtowicz, K. & Zabel, M. The role of aldehyde dehydrogenase (ALDH) in cancer drug resistance. *Biomedicine & Pharmacotherapy* **67**, 669-680 (2013).

33.   D'Alterio, C., Scala, S., Sozzi, G., Roz, L. & Bertolini, G. Paradoxical effects of chemotherapy on tumor relapse and metastasis promotion. *Seminars in Cancer Biology* **60**, 351-361 (2020).

34.   Duesberg, P., Stindl, R. & Hehlmann, R. Explaining the high mutation rates of cancer cells to drug and multidrug resistance by chromosome reassortments that are catalyzed by aneuploidy. *Proc Natl Acad Sci U S A* **97**, 14295-14300 (2000).

35.   Ji, X., *et al.* Chemoresistance mechanisms of breast cancer and their countermeasures. *Biomedicine & Pharmacotherapy* **114**, 108800 (2019).

36.   Chen, Y., *et al.* Twist confers chemoresistance to anthracyclines in bladder cancer through upregulating P-glycoprotein. *Chemotherapy* **58**, 264-272 (2012).

37.   Bao, L., *et al.* Increased expression of P-glycoprotein and doxorubicin chemoresistance of metastatic breast cancer is regulated by miR-298. *The American journal of pathology* **180**, 2490-2503 (2012).

38.   Robinson, K. & Tiriveedhi, V. Perplexing Role of P-Glycoprotein in Tumor Microenvironment. *Frontiers in Oncology* **10**(2020).

39.   Townsend, D.M. & Tew, K.D. The role of glutathione-S-transferase in anti-cancer drug resistance. *Oncogene* **22**, 7369-7375 (2003).

40.   Traverso, N., *et al.* Role of Glutathione in Cancer Progression and Chemoresistance. *Oxidative Medicine and Cellular Longevity* **2013**, 972913 (2013).

41.   Carretero, J., *et al.* Growth-associated changes in glutathione content correlate with liver metastatic activity of B16 melanoma cells. *Clinical & Experimental Metastasis* **17**, 567 (1999).

42.   Rodriguez-Torres, M. & Allan, A.L. Aldehyde dehydrogenase as a marker and functional mediator of metastasis in solid tumors. *Clinical & experimental metastasis* **33**, 97-113 (2016).

43.   Karagiannis, G.S., Condeelis, J.S. & Oktay, M.H. Chemotherapy-Induced Metastasis: Molecular Mechanisms, Clinical Manifestations, Therapeutic Interventions. *Cancer Res* **79**, 4567 (2019).

44.   Chen, W.J., *et al.* Cancer-associated fibroblasts regulate the plasticity of lung cancer stemness via paracrine signalling. *Nat Commun* **5**(2014).

45.   Acharyya, S., *et al.* A CXCL1 paracrine network links cancer chemoresistance and metastasis. *Cell* **150**, 165-178 (2012).

46.   Obenauf, A.C., *et al.* Therapy-induced tumour secretomes promote resistance and tumour progression. *Nature* **520**, 368-372 (2015).

47.   Alluri, P.G., Speers, C. & Chinnaiyan, A.M. Estrogen receptor mutations and their role in breast cancer progression. *Breast Cancer Res* **16**, 494-494 (2014).

48.   Blomberg, O.S., Spagnuolo, L. & de Visser, K.E. Immune regulation of metastasis: mechanistic insights and therapeutic opportunities. *Dis Model Mech* **11**, dmm036236 (2018).

49.   Lengagne, R., *et al.* Distinct role for CD8 T cells toward cutaneous tumors and visceral metastases. *J Immunol* **180**, 130-137 (2008).

50.   Eyles, J., *et al.* Tumor cells disseminate early, but immunosurveillance limits metastatic outgrowth, in a mouse model of melanoma. *J Clin Invest* **120**, 2030-2039 (2010).

51.   Takeda, K., *et al.* Involvement of tumor necrosis factor-related apoptosis-inducing ligand in surveillance of tumor metastasis by liver natural killer cells. *Nat Med* **7**, 94-100 (2001).

52.   López-Soto, A., Gonzalez, S., Smyth, M.J. & Galluzzi, L. Control of Metastasis by NK Cells. *Cancer Cell* **32**, 135-154 (2017).

53.   Mahmoud, S.M., *et al.* Tumor-infiltrating CD8+ lymphocytes predict clinical outcome in breast cancer. *J Clin Oncol* **29**, 1949-1955 (2011).

54.   Galon, J., *et al.* Type, density, and location of immune cells within human colorectal tumors predict clinical outcome. *Science* **313**, 1960-1964 (2006).

55.   Huh, J.W., Lee, J.H. & Kim, H.R. Prognostic Significance of Tumor-Infiltrating Lymphocytes for Patients With Colorectal Cancer. *Archives of Surgery* **147**, 366-372 (2012).

56.   Zhang, L., *et al.* Intratumoral T cells, recurrence, and survival in epithelial ovarian cancer. *N Engl J Med* **348**, 203-213 (2003).

57.   Olkhanud, P.B., *et al.* Breast cancer lung metastasis requires expression of chemokine receptor CCR4 and regulatory T cells. *Cancer Res* **69**, 5996-6004 (2009).

58.   Smyth, M.J., *et al.* Differential tumor surveillance by natural killer (NK) and NKT cells. *The Journal of experimental medicine* **191**, 661-668 (2000).

59.   Fridlender, Z.G., *et al.* Polarization of tumor-associated neutrophil phenotype by TGF-beta: "N1" versus "N2" TAN. *Cancer Cell* **16**, 183-194 (2009).

60.   Flavell, R.A., Sanjabi, S., Wrzesinski, S.H. & Licona-Limón, P. The polarization of immune cells in the tumour environment by TGFbeta. *Nat Rev Immunol* **10**, 554-567 (2010).

61.   Mantovani, A., Sozzani, S., Locati, M., Allavena, P. & Sica, A. Macrophage polarization: tumor-associated macrophages as a paradigm for polarized M2 mononuclear phagocytes. *Trends Immunol* **23**, 549-555 (2002).

62.   Ondondo, B., Jones, E., Godkin, A. & Gallimore, A. Home sweet home: the tumor microenvironment as a haven for regulatory T cells. *Front Immunol* **4**, 197 (2013).

63.   Coffelt, S.B., *et al.* IL-17-producing γδ T cells and neutrophils conspire to promote breast cancer metastasis. *Nature* **522**, 345-348 (2015).

64.   DeNardo, D.G., *et al.* CD4(+) T cells regulate pulmonary metastasis of mammary carcinomas by enhancing protumor properties of macrophages. *Cancer Cell* **16**, 91-102 (2009).

65.   Henke, E., Nandigama, R. & Ergün, S. Extracellular Matrix in the Tumor Microenvironment and Its Impact on Cancer Therapy. *Front Mol Biosci* **6**, 160-160 (2020).

66.   Castermans, K. & Griffioen, A.W. Tumor blood vessels, a difficult hurdle for infiltrating leukocytes. *Biochimica et Biophysica Acta (BBA) - Reviews on Cancer* **1776**, 160-174 (2007).

67.   He, X. & Xu, C. Immune checkpoint signaling and cancer immunotherapy. *Cell Research* **30**, 660-669 (2020).

68.   Iwai, Y., *et al.* Involvement of PD-L1 on tumor cells in the escape from host immune system and tumor immunotherapy by PD-L1 blockade. *Proc Natl Acad Sci U S A* **99**, 12293-12297 (2002).

69.   Syn, N.L., Teng, M.W.L., Mok, T.S.K. & Soo, R.A. De-novo and acquired resistance to immune checkpoint targeting. *The Lancet Oncology* **18**, e731-e741 (2017).

70.   Schmid, P., *et al.* Atezolizumab and Nab-Paclitaxel in Advanced Triple-Negative Breast Cancer. *New England Journal of Medicine* **379**, 2108-2121 (2018).

71.   Szekely, B., *et al.* Immunological differences between primary and metastatic breast cancer. *Annals of Oncology* **29**, 2232-2239 (2018).

72.   Planes-Laine, G., *et al.* PD-1/PD-L1 Targeting in Breast Cancer: The First Clinical Evidences Are Emerging. A Literature Review. *Cancers (Basel)* **11**, 1033 (2019).

73.   June, C.H. & Sadelain, M. Chimeric Antigen Receptor Therapy. *N Engl J Med* **379**, 64-73 (2018).

74.   Bagley, S.J. & O'Rourke, D.M. Clinical investigation of CAR T cells for solid tumors: Lessons learned and future directions. *Pharmacology & Therapeutics* **205**, 107419 (2020).

75.   Anderson, N.R., Minutolo, N.G., Gill, S. & Klichinsky, M. Macrophage-Based Approaches for Cancer Immunotherapy. *Cancer Res* **81**, 1201 (2021).

76.   Pienta, K.J., *et al.* Phase 2 study of carlumab (CNTO 888), a human monoclonal antibody against CC-chemokine ligand 2 (CCL2), in metastatic castration-resistant prostate cancer. *Invest New Drugs* **31**, 760-768 (2013).

77.   Advani, R., *et al.* CD47 Blockade by Hu5F9-G4 and Rituximab in Non-Hodgkin's Lymphoma. *New England Journal of Medicine* **379**, 1711-1721 (2018).

78.   Jahchan, N.S., *et al.* Tuning the Tumor Myeloid Microenvironment to Fight Cancer. *Front Immunol* **10**(2019).

79.   Sandhu, S.K., *et al.* A first-in-human, first-in-class, phase I study of carlumab (CNTO 888), a human monoclonal antibody against CC-chemokine ligand 2 in patients with solid tumors. *Cancer Chemotherapy and Pharmacology* **71**, 1041-1050 (2013).

80.   Bonapace, L., *et al.* Cessation of CCL2 inhibition accelerates breast cancer metastasis by promoting angiogenesis. *Nature* **515**, 130-133 (2014).

81.   Cha, Y.J. & Koo, J.S. Role of Tumor-Associated Myeloid Cells in Breast Cancer. *Cells* **9**, 1785 (2020).

82.   Janni, W., *et al.* Abstract GS1-06: Extended adjuvant bisphosphonate treatment over five years in early breast cancer does not improve disease-free and overall survival compared to two years of treatment: Phase III data from the SUCCESS A study. *Cancer Res* **78**, GS1-06 (2018).

83.   Gnant, M. Zoledronic acid in breast cancer: latest findings and interpretations. *Ther Adv Med Oncol* **3**, 293-301 (2011).

84.   Law, A.M.K., Valdes-Mora, F. & Gallego-Ortega, D. Myeloid-Derived Suppressor Cells as a Therapeutic Target for Cancer. *Cells* **9**, 561 (2020).

85.   Metzler, J.M., Burla, L., Fink, D. & Imesch, P. Ibrutinib in Gynecological Malignancies and Breast Cancer: A Systematic Review. *Int J Mol Sci* **21**, 4154 (2020).

86.   Varikuti, S., *et al.* Ibrutinib treatment inhibits breast cancer progression and metastasis by inducing conversion of myeloid-derived suppressor cells to dendritic cells. *Br J Cancer* **122**, 1005-1013 (2020).

87.   Sagiv-Barfi, I., *et al.* Therapeutic antitumor immunity by checkpoint blockade is enhanced by ibrutinib, an inhibitor of both BTK and ITK. *Proc Natl Acad Sci U S A* **112**, E966-E972 (2015).

88.   Hong, D., *et al.* A Phase 1b/2 Study of the Bruton Tyrosine Kinase Inhibitor Ibrutinib and the PD-L1 Inhibitor Durvalumab in Patients with Pretreated Solid Tumors. *Oncology* **97**, 102-111 (2019).

89.   Guo, F.F. & Cui, J.W. The Role of Tumor-Infiltrating B Cells in Tumor Immunity. *J Oncol* **2019**, 2592419-2592419 (2019).

90.   Garaud, S., *et al.* Tumor infiltrating B-cells signal functional humoral immune responses in breast cancer. *JCI Insight* **5**, e129641 (2019).

91.   Pieper, K., Grimbacher, B. & Eibel, H. B-cell biology and development. *Journal of Allergy and Clinical Immunology* **131**, 959-971 (2013).

92.   Largeot, A., Pagano, G., Gonder, S., Moussay, E. & Paggetti, J. The B-side of Cancer Immunity: The Underrated Tune. *Cells* **8**, 449 (2019).

93.   Wortman, J.C., *et al.* Spatial distribution of B cells and lymphocyte clusters as a predictor of triple-negative breast cancer outcome. *npj Breast Cancer* **7**, 84 (2021).

94.   Alsughayyir, J., Pettigrew, G.J. & Motallebzadeh, R. Spoiling for a Fight: B Lymphocytes As Initiator and Effector Populations within Tertiary Lymphoid Organs in Autoimmunity and Transplantation. *Front Immunol* **8**, 1639-1639 (2017).

95.   Peske, J.D., *et al.* Effector lymphocyte-induced lymph node-like vasculature enables naive T-cell entry into tumours and enhanced anti-tumour immunity. *Nat Commun* **6**, 7114-7114 (2015).

96.   Zhu, G., *et al.* Induction of Tertiary Lymphoid Structures With Antitumor Function by a Lymph Node-Derived Stromal Cell Line. *Front Immunol* **9**, 1609-1609 (2018).

97.   Castino, G.F., *et al.* Spatial distribution of B cells predicts prognosis in human pancreatic adenocarcinoma. *Oncoimmunology* **5**, e1085147-e1085147 (2015).

98.   Yu, H.-M., Yang, J.-L., Jiao, S.-C. & Wang, J.-D. [Prognostic value of B lymphocyte infiltration in breast cancer.]. *Nan fang yi ke da xue xue bao = Journal of Southern Medical University* **33**, 750-755 (2013).

99.   Garg, K., *et al.* Tumor-associated B cells in cutaneous primary melanoma and improved clinical outcome. *Human Pathology* **54**, 157-164 (2016).

100.   Sakimura, C., *et al.* B cells in tertiary lymphoid structures are associated with favorable prognosis in gastric cancer. *Journal of Surgical Research* **215**, 74-82 (2017).

101.   Hennequin, A., *et al.* Tumor infiltration by Tbet+ effector T cells and CD20+ B cells is associated with survival in gastric cancer patients. *Oncoimmunology* **5**, e1054598-e1054598 (2015).

102.   Nielsen, J.S., *et al.* CD20⁺ Tumor-Infiltrating Lymphocytes Have an Atypical CD27[−] Memory Phenotype and Together with CD8⁺ T Cells Promote Favorable Prognosis in Ovarian Cancer. *Clinical Cancer Research* **18**, 3281 (2012).

103.   Dong, H.P., *et al.* NK- and B-Cell Infiltration Correlates With Worse Outcome in Metastatic Ovarian Carcinoma. *American Journal of Clinical Pathology* **125**, 451-458 (2006).

104.   Kroeger, D.R., Milne, K. & Nelson, B.H. Tumor-Infiltrating Plasma Cells Are Associated with Tertiary Lymphoid Structures, Cytolytic T-Cell Responses, and Superior Prognosis in Ovarian Cancer. *Clinical Cancer Research* **22**, 3005 (2016).

105.   Dieu-Nosjean, M.-C., *et al.* Long-Term Survival for Patients With Non–Small-Cell Lung Cancer With Intratumoral Lymphoid Structures. *Journal of Clinical Oncology* **26**, 4410-4417 (2008).

106.   Calderaro, J., *et al.* Intra-tumoral tertiary lymphoid structures are associated with a low risk of early recurrence of hepatocellular carcinoma. *Journal of Hepatology* **70**, 58-65 (2019).

107.   Wada, Y., Nakashima, O., Kutami, R., Yamamoto, O. & Kojiro, M. Clinicopathological study on hepatocellular carcinoma with lymphocytic infiltration. *Hepatology* **27**, 407-414 (1998).

108.   Behr, D.S., *et al.* Prognostic value of immune cell infiltration, tertiary lymphoid structures and PD-L1 expression in Merkel cell carcinomas. *Int J Clin Exp Pathol* **7**, 7610-7621 (2014).

109.   Jiang, Q., *et al.* CD19+ tumor-infiltrating B-cells prime CD4+ T-cell immunity and predict platinum-based chemotherapy efficacy in muscle-invasive bladder cancer. *Cancer Immunology, Immunotherapy* **68**, 45-56 (2019).

110.   Coppola, D., *et al.* Unique ectopic lymph node-like structures present in human primary colorectal carcinoma are identified by immune gene array profiling. *The American journal of pathology* **179**, 37-45 (2011).

111.   Bergomas, F., *et al.* Tertiary intratumor lymphoid tissue in colo-rectal cancer. *Cancers (Basel)* **4**, 1-10 (2011).

112.   Shah, S., *et al.* Increased rejection of primary tumors in mice lacking B cells: Inhibition of anti-tumor CTL and TH1 cytokine responses by B cells. *Int J Cancer* **117**, 574-586 (2005).

113. Coronella-Wood, J.A. & Hersh, E.M. Naturally occurring B-cell responses to breast cancer. *Cancer Immunology, Immunotherapy* **52**, 715-738 (2003).

114. de Visser, K.E., Korets, L.V. & Coussens, L.M. De novo carcinogenesis promoted by chronic inflammation is B lymphocyte dependent. *Cancer Cell* **7**, 411-423 (2005).

115. de Visser, K.E., Eichten, A. & Coussens, L.M. Paradoxical roles of the immune system during cancer development. *Nature Reviews Cancer* **6**, 24-37 (2006).

116. Lee, K.E., *et al.* Hif1a Deletion Reveals Pro-Neoplastic Function of B Cells in Pancreatic Neoplasia. *Cancer discovery* **6**, 256-269 (2016).

117. Pylayeva-Gupta, Y., *et al.* IL35-Producing B Cells Promote the Development of Pancreatic Neoplasia. *Cancer discovery* **6**, 247-255 (2016).

118. Schioppa, T., *et al.* B regulatory cells and the tumor-promoting actions of TNF-α during squamous carcinogenesis. *Proceedings of the National Academy of Sciences* **108**, 10662 (2011).

119. Zhou, X., Su, Y.-X., Lao, X.-M., Liang, Y.-J. & Liao, G.-Q. CD19+IL-10+ regulatory B cells affect survival of tongue squamous cell carcinoma patients and induce resting CD4+ T cells to CD4+Foxp3+ regulatory T cells. *Oral Oncology* **53**, 27-35 (2016).

120. Guan, H., *et al.* PD-L1 mediated the differentiation of tumor-infiltrating CD19(+) B lymphocytes and T cells in Invasive breast cancer. *Oncoimmunology* **5**, e1075112-e1075112 (2015).

121. Lelekakis, M., *et al.* A novel orthotopic model of breast cancer metastasis to bone. *Clinical & Experimental Metastasis* **17**, 163-170 (1999).

122. Pulaski, B.A. & Ostrand-Rosenberg, S. Mouse 4T1 Breast Tumor Model. *Current Protocols in Immunology* **39**, 20.22.21-20.22.16 (2000).

123. Olkhanud, P.B., *et al.* Tumor-evoked regulatory B cells promote breast cancer metastasis by converting resting CD4+ T cells to T-regulatory cells. *Cancer Res* **71**, 3505-3515 (2011).

124. Zhang, Y., *et al.* B lymphocyte inhibition of anti-tumor response depends on expansion of Treg but is independent of B-cell IL-10 secretion. *Cancer Immunology, Immunotherapy* **62**, 87-99 (2013).

125. Zhang, Y., Morgan, R., Podack, E.R. & Rosenblatt, J. B cell regulation of anti-tumor immune response. *Immunologic Research* **57**, 115-124 (2013).

126. Bodogai, M., *et al.* Anti-CD20 antibody promotes cancer escape via enrichment of tumor-evoked regulatory B cells expressing low levels of CD20 and CD137L. *Cancer Res* **73**, 2127-2138 (2013).

127.   Tan, T.-T. & Coussens, L.M. Humoral immunity, inflammation and cancer. *Current Opinion in Immunology* **19**, 209-216 (2007).

128.   Dass, T.K., Aziz, M., Rattan, A. & Tyagi, S.P. Clinical utility and monitoring of breast cancer by circulating immune complexes. *Indian journal of pathology & microbiology* **35**, 298-307 (1992).

129.   Nakahara, T., Norberg, S.M., Shalinsky, D.R., Hu-Lowe, D.D. & McDonald, D.M. Effect of Inhibition of Vascular Endothelial Growth Factor Signaling on Distribution of Extravasated Antibodies in Tumors. *Cancer Res* **66**, 1434 (2006).

130.   Barbera-Guillem, E., May, K.F., Nyhus, J.K. & Nelson, M.B. Promotion of Tumor Invasion by Cooperation of Granulocytes and Macrophages Activated by Anti-tumor Antibodies. *Neoplasia* **1**, 453-460 (1999).

131.   Gu, Y., *et al.* Tumor-educated B cells selectively promote breast cancer lymph node metastasis by HSPA4-targeting IgG. *Nature Medicine* **25**, 312-322 (2019).

132.   Hanahan, D. & Weinberg, R.A. Hallmarks of cancer: the next generation. *Cell* **144**, 646-674 (2011).

133.   Fearon, K.C., Glass, D.J. & Guttridge, D.C. Cancer cachexia: mediators, signaling, and metabolic pathways. *Cell Metab* **16**, 153-166 (2012).

134.   Biswas, A.K. & Acharyya, S. Cancer-Associated Cachexia: A Systemic Consequence of Cancer Progression. *Annual Review of Cancer Biology* **4**, 391-411 (2020).

135.   Argilés, J.M., Busquets, S. & López-Soriano, F.J. Cancer cachexia, a clinical challenge. *Curr Opin Oncol* **31**, 286-290 (2019).

136.   Loberg, R.D., Bradley, D.A., Tomlins, S.A., Chinnaiyan, A.M. & Pienta, K.J. The Lethal Phenotype of Cancer: The Molecular Basis of Death Due to Malignancy. *CA: A Cancer Journal for Clinicians* **57**, 225-241 (2007).

137.   Fearon, K., *et al.* Definition and classification of cancer cachexia: an international consensus. *The Lancet Oncology* **12**, 489-495 (2011).

138.   Chan, D.S.M., *et al.* Body mass index and survival in women with breast cancer-systematic literature review and meta-analysis of 82 follow-up studies. *Ann Oncol* **25**, 1901-1914 (2014).

139.   Kwan, M.L., *et al.* Pre-diagnosis body mass index and survival after breast cancer in the After Breast Cancer Pooling Project. *Breast cancer research and treatment* **132**, 729-739 (2012).

140.   Bruera, E. & Sweeney, C. Cachexia and asthenia in cancer patients. *The Lancet Oncology* **1**, 138-147 (2000).

141.   Argiles, J.M., Busquets, S., Stemmler, B. & Lopez-Soriano, F.J. Cancer cachexia: understanding the molecular basis. *Nature reviews. Cancer* **14**, 754-762 (2014).

142.   Bachmann, J., *et al.* Cachexia Worsens Prognosis in Patients with Resectable Pancreatic Cancer. *Journal of Gastrointestinal Surgery* **12**, 1193 (2008).

143.   Kalantar-Zadeh, K., *et al.* Why cachexia kills: examining the causality of poor outcomes in wasting conditions. *J Cachexia Sarcopenia Muscle* **4**, 89-94 (2013).

144.   Damrauer, J.S., *et al.* Chemotherapy-induced muscle wasting: association with NF-κB and cancer cachexia. *Eur J Transl Myol* **28**, 7590-7590 (2018).

145.   Barreto, R., *et al.* Chemotherapy-related cachexia is associated with mitochondrial depletion and the activation of ERK1/2 and p38 MAPKs. *Oncotarget* **7**, 43442-43460 (2016).

146.   Acharyya, S. & Guttridge, D.C. Cancer Cachexia Signaling Pathways Continue to Emerge Yet Much Still Points to the Proteasome. *Clinical Cancer Research* **13**, 1356 (2007).

147.   Morley, J.E., Thomas, D.R. & Wilson, M.-M.G. Cachexia: pathophysiology and clinical relevance. *The American Journal of Clinical Nutrition* **83**, 735-743 (2006).

148.   Ali, S. & Garcia, J.M. Sarcopenia, Cachexia and Aging: Diagnosis, Mechanisms and Therapeutic Options - A Mini-Review. *Gerontology* **60**, 294-305 (2014).

149.   Tomasin, R., Martin, A.C.B.M. & Cominetti, M.R. Metastasis and cachexia: alongside in clinics, but not so in animal models. *J Cachexia Sarcopenia Muscle* **10**, 1183-1194 (2019).

150.   Ni, X., Yang, J. & Li, M. Imaging-guided curative surgical resection of pancreatic cancer in a xenograft mouse model. *Cancer Lett* **324**, 179-185 (2012).

151.   Norton, J.A., Moley, J.F., Green, M.V., Carson, R.E. & Morrison, S.D. Parabiotic Transfer of Cancer Anorexia/Cachexia in Male Rats. *Cancer Res* **45**, 5547 (1985).

152.   Argilés, J.M., Stemmler, B., López-Soriano, F.J. & Busquets, S. Nonmuscle Tissues Contribution to Cancer Cachexia. *Mediators Inflamm* **2015**, 182872-182872 (2015).

153.   Biswas, A.K. & Acharyya, S. Understanding cachexia in the context of metastatic progression. *Nature Reviews Cancer* **20**, 274-284 (2020).

154.   Montano, M. 6 - Translational models, methods and concepts in studies of muscle tissue repair. in *Translational Biology in Medicine* (ed. Montano, M.) 103-128 (Woodhead Publishing, 2014).

155.   Cai, D., *et al.* IKKbeta/NF-kappaB activation causes severe muscle wasting in mice. *Cell* **119**, 285-298 (2004).

156. Guttridge, D.C., Mayo, M.W., Madrid, L.V., Wang, C.-Y. & Baldwin Jr, A.S. NF-κB-Induced Loss of <em>MyoD</em> Messenger RNA: Possible Role in Muscle Decay and Cachexia. *Science* **289**, 2363 (2000).

157. Fukawa, T., *et al.* Excessive fatty acid oxidation induces muscle atrophy in cancer cachexia. *Nat Med* **22**, 666-671 (2016).

158. Zhang, G., *et al.* Tumor induces muscle wasting in mice through releasing extracellular Hsp70 and Hsp90. *Nat Commun* **8**, 589-589 (2017).

159. He, W.A., *et al.* Microvesicles containing miRNAs promote muscle cell death in cancer cachexia via TLR7. *Proc Natl Acad Sci U S A* **111**, 4525-4529 (2014).

160. Petruzzelli, M., *et al.* A switch from white to brown fat increases energy expenditure in cancer-associated cachexia. *Cell Metab* **20**, 433-447 (2014).

161. Baracos, V.E., Martin, L., Korc, M., Guttridge, D.C. & Fearon, K.C.H. Cancer-associated cachexia. *Nature Reviews Disease Primers* **4**, 17105 (2018).

162. Jeong, J. & Eide, D.J. The SLC39 family of zinc transporters. *Molecular aspects of medicine* **34**, 612-619 (2013).

163. Maret, W. & Sandstead, H.H. Zinc requirements and the risks and benefits of zinc supplementation. *J Trace Elem Med Biol* **20**, 3-18 (2006).

164. Lu, J., Stewart, A.J., Sadler, P.J., Pinheiro, T.J. & Blindauer, C.A. Albumin as a zinc carrier: properties of its high-affinity zinc-binding site. *Biochem Soc Trans* **36**, 1317-1321 (2008).

165. Siren, P.M. & Siren, M.J. Systemic zinc redistribution and dyshomeostasis in cancer cachexia. *J Cachexia Sarcopenia Muscle* **1**, 23-33 (2010).

166. Fabris, C., *et al.* Copper, zinc and copper/zinc ratio in chronic pancreatitis and pancreatic cancer. *Clinical Biochemistry* **18**, 373-375 (1985).

167. Wang, Y., Sun, Z., Li, A. & Zhang, Y. Association between serum zinc levels and lung cancer: a meta-analysis of observational studies. *World Journal of Surgical Oncology* **17**, 78 (2019).

168. Al-Ansari, R.F., Al-Gebori, A.M. & Sulaiman, G.M. Serum levels of zinc, copper, selenium and glutathione peroxidase in the different groups of colorectal cancer patients. *Caspian J Intern Med* **11**, 384-390 (2020).

169. Larsson, S., Karlberg, I., Selin, E., Daneryd, P. & Peterson, H.I. Trace element changes in serum and skeletal muscle compared to tumour tissue in sarcoma-bearing rats. *In Vivo* **1**, 131-140 (1987).

170.   Russell, S.T., Siren, P.M., Siren, M.J. & Tisdale, M.J. The role of zinc in the anti-tumour and anti-cachectic activity of D-myo-inositol 1,2,6-triphosphate. *Br J Cancer* **102**, 833-836 (2010).

171.   Wang, G., *et al.* Metastatic cancers promote cachexia through ZIP14 upregulation in skeletal muscle. *Nature Medicine* **24**, 770-781 (2018).

172.   Stark, A.P., *et al.* Long-term survival in patients with pancreatic ductal adenocarcinoma. *Surgery* **159**, 1520-1527 (2016).

173.   Howlader N, N.A., Krapcho M, Miller D, Brest A, Yu M, Ruhl J, Tatalovich Z, Mariotto A, Lewis DR, Chen HS, Feuer EJ, Cronin KA (eds). SEER Cancer Statistics Review, 1975-2018. *National Cancer Institute. Bethesda, MD* **https://seer.cancer.gov/csr/1975_2018/, based on November 2020 SEER data submission, posted to the SEER web site, April 2021.**

174.   Rawla, P., Sunkara, T. & Gaduputi, V. Epidemiology of Pancreatic Cancer: Global Trends, Etiology and Risk Factors. *World journal of oncology* **10**, 10-27 (2019).

175.   Henderson, S.E., Makhijani, N. & Mace, T.A. Pancreatic Cancer-Induced Cachexia and Relevant Mouse Models. *Pancreas* **47**, 937-945 (2018).

176.   Adamska, A., Domenichini, A. & Falasca, M. Pancreatic Ductal Adenocarcinoma: Current and Evolving Therapies. *Int J Mol Sci* **18**(2017).

177.   Sohn, T.A., *et al.* Resected adenocarcinoma of the pancreas—616 patients: results, outcomes, and prognostic indicators. *Journal of Gastrointestinal Surgery* **4**, 567-579 (2000).

178.   Greco, S.H., *et al.* TGF-beta Blockade Reduces Mortality and Metabolic Changes in a Validated Murine Model of Pancreatic Cancer Cachexia. *PLoS One* **10**, e0132786 (2015).

179.   Corbett, T.H., *et al.* Induction and Chemotherapeutic Response of Two Transplantable Ductal Adenocarcinomas of the Pancreas in C57BL/6 Mice. *Cancer Res* **44**, 717 (1984).

180.   Aydemir, T.B. & Cousins, R.J. The Multiple Faces of the Metal Transporter ZIP14 (SLC39A14). *The Journal of nutrition* **148**, 174-184 (2018).

181.   Lichten, L.A. & Cousins, R.J. Mammalian Zinc Transporters: Nutritional and Physiologic Regulation. *Annual Review of Nutrition* **29**, 153-176 (2009).

182.   Li, M., *et al.* Aberrant expression of zinc transporter ZIP4 (SLC39A4) significantly contributes to human pancreatic cancer pathogenesis and progression. *Proceedings of the National Academy of Sciences of the United States of America* **104**, 18636-18641 (2007).

183.   Hendifar, A.E., *et al.* Pancreas Cancer-Associated Weight Loss. *Oncologist* **24**, 691-701 (2019).

184.   Roberts, B.M., *et al.* Diaphragm and ventilatory dysfunction during cancer cachexia. *FASEB J* **27**, 2600-2610 (2013).

185.   Shakri, A.R., *et al.* Upregulation of ZIP14 and Altered Zinc Homeostasis in Muscles in Pancreatic Cancer Cachexia. *Cancers (Basel)* **12**(2020).

186.   Daley, D., *et al.* γδ T Cells Support Pancreatic Oncogenesis by Restraining αβ T Cell Activation. *Cell* **166**, 1485-1499.e1415 (2016).

187.   Moo-Young, T.A., *et al.* Tumor-derived TGF-beta mediates conversion of CD4+Foxp3+ regulatory T cells in a murine model of pancreas cancer. *J Immunother* **32**, 12-21 (2009).

188.   Pilon-Thomas, S., *et al.* Murine pancreatic adenocarcinoma dampens SHIP-1 expression and alters MDSC homeostasis and function. *PLoS One* **6**, e27729-e27729 (2011).

189.   Zhao, J., *et al.* Clinical and prognostic significance of serum transforming growth factor-beta1 levels in patients with pancreatic ductal adenocarcinoma. *Braz J Med Biol Res* **49**, e5485 (2016).

190.   Yu, Z., *et al.* Zinc chelator TPEN induces pancreatic cancer cell death through causing oxidative stress and inhibiting cell autophagy. *Journal of cellular physiology* **234**, 20648-20661 (2019).

191.   Hashemi, M., Ghavami, S., Eshraghi, M., Booy, E.P. & Los, M. Cytotoxic effects of intra and extracellular zinc chelation on human breast cancer cells. *European journal of pharmacology* **557**, 9-19 (2007).

192.   Mendivil-Perez, M., Velez-Pardo, C. & Jimenez-Del-Rio, M. TPEN induces apoptosis independently of zinc chelator activity in a model of acute lymphoblastic leukemia and ex vivo acute leukemia cells through oxidative stress and mitochondria caspase-3- and AIF-dependent pathways. *Oxid Med Cell Longev* **2012**, 313275 (2012).

193.   Habel, N., *et al.* Zinc chelation: a metallothionein 2A's mechanism of action involved in osteosarcoma cell death and chemotherapy resistance. *Cell death & disease* **4**, e874 (2013).

194.   Makhov, P., *et al.* Zinc chelation induces rapid depletion of the X-linked inhibitor of apoptosis and sensitizes prostate cancer cells to TRAIL-mediated apoptosis. *Cell death and differentiation* **15**, 1745-1751 (2008).

195.   Zuo, J., *et al.* Novel Polypyridyl chelators deplete cellular zinc and destabilize the X-linked inhibitor of apoptosis protein (XIAP) prior to induction of apoptosis in human prostate and breast cancer cells. *Journal of cellular biochemistry* **113**, 2567-2575 (2012).

196.   Stuart, C.H., *et al.* Prostate-specific membrane antigen-targeted liposomes specifically deliver the Zn(2+) chelator TPEN inducing oxidative stress in prostate cancer cells. *Nanomedicine (Lond)* **11**, 1207-1222 (2016).

197. Prado, C.M. & Heymsfield, S.B. Lean tissue imaging: a new era for nutritional assessment and intervention. *JPEN J Parenter Enteral Nutr* **38**, 940-953 (2014).

198. Prado, C.M., *et al.* Sarcopenia and physical function in overweight patients with advanced cancer. *Can J Diet Pract Res* **74**, 69-74 (2013).

199. Di Sebastiano, K.M. & Mourtzakis, M. A critical evaluation of body composition modalities used to assess adipose and skeletal muscle tissue in cancer. *Appl Physiol Nutr Metab* **37**, 811-821 (2012).

200. Shang, L., *et al.* Impact of post-diagnosis weight change on survival outcomes in Black and White breast cancer patients. *Breast Cancer Research* **23**, 18 (2021).

201. Balmaña, J., Díez, O., Rubio, I.T. & Cardoso, F. BRCA in breast cancer: ESMO Clinical Practice Guidelines. *Annals of Oncology* **22**, vi31-vi34 (2011).

202. Geenen, J.J.J., Linn, S.C., Beijnen, J.H. & Schellens, J.H.M. PARP Inhibitors in the Treatment of Triple-Negative Breast Cancer. *Clinical Pharmacokinetics* **57**, 427-437 (2018).

203. Greenup, R., *et al.* Prevalence of BRCA Mutations Among Women with Triple-Negative Breast Cancer (TNBC) in a Genetic Counseling Cohort. *Annals of Surgical Oncology* **20**, 3254-3258 (2013).

204. Huszno, J., Kołosza, Z. & Grzybowska, E. BRCA1 mutation in breast cancer patients: Analysis of prognostic factors and survival. *Oncol Lett* **17**, 1986-1995 (2019).

205. Wu, L.C., *et al.* Identification of a RING protein that can interact in vivo with the BRCA1 gene product. *Nature Genetics* **14**, 430-440 (1996).

206. Jiang, Q. & Greenberg, R.A. Deciphering the BRCA1 Tumor Suppressor Network. *J Biol Chem* **290**, 17724-17732 (2015).

207. Ludwig, T., Fisher, P., Ganesan, S. & Efstratiadis, A. Tumorigenesis in mice carrying a truncating Brca1 mutation. *Genes Dev* **15**, 1188-1193 (2001).

208. Shakya, R., *et al.* The basal-like mammary carcinomas induced by <em>Brca1</em> or <em>Bard1</em> inactivation implicate the BRCA1/BARD1 heterodimer in tumor suppression. *Proceedings of the National Academy of Sciences* **105**, 7040 (2008).

209. Baer, R. & Ludwig, T. The BRCA1/BARD1 heterodimer, a tumor suppressor complex with ubiquitin E3 ligase activity. *Curr Opin Genet Dev* **12**, 86-91 (2002).

210. Keung, Y.T.M., Wu, Y. & Vadgama, V.J. PARP Inhibitors as a Therapeutic Agent for Homologous Recombination Deficiency in Breast Cancers. *Journal of Clinical Medicine* **8**(2019).

211.   Pilie, P.G., Tang, C., Mills, G.B. & Yap, T.A. State-of-the-art strategies for targeting the DNA damage response in cancer. *Nat Rev Clin Oncol* **16**, 81-104 (2019).

212.   Byrum, A.K., Vindigni, A. & Mosammaparast, N. Defining and Modulating 'BRCAness'. *Trends Cell Biol* **29**, 740-751 (2019).

213.   Chacon-Cabrera, A., *et al.* Role of PARP activity in lung cancer-induced cachexia: Effects on muscle oxidative stress, proteolysis, anabolic markers, and phenotype. *Journal of cellular physiology* **232**, 3744-3761 (2017).

214.   DeSantis, C.E., *et al.* Breast cancer statistics, 2019. *CA: A Cancer Journal for Clinicians* **69**, 438-451 (2019).

215.   Redig, A.J. & McAllister, S.S. Breast cancer as a systemic disease: a view of metastasis. *J Intern Med* **274**, 113-126 (2013).

216.   Garrido-Castro, A.C., Lin, N.U. & Polyak, K. Insights into Molecular Classifications of Triple-Negative Breast Cancer: Improving Patient Selection for Treatment. *Cancer Discovery* **9**, 176 (2019).

217.   Aysola, K., *et al.* Triple Negative Breast Cancer - An Overview. *Hereditary Genet* **2013**, 001 (2013).

218.   Dent, R., *et al.* Triple-Negative Breast Cancer: Clinical Features and Patterns of Recurrence. *Clinical Cancer Research* **13**, 4429 (2007).

219.   Wu, Q., *et al.* Breast cancer subtypes predict the preferential site of distant metastases: a SEER based study. *Oncotarget* **8**, 27990-27996 (2017).

220.   Kassam, F., *et al.* Survival Outcomes for Patients with Metastatic Triple-Negative Breast Cancer: Implications for Clinical Practice and Trial Design. *Clinical Breast Cancer* **9**, 29-33 (2009).

221.   Echeverria, G.V., *et al.* Resistance to neoadjuvant chemotherapy in triple-negative breast cancer mediated by a reversible drug-tolerant state. *Sci Transl Med* **11**, eaav0936 (2019).

222.   Symmans, W.F., *et al.* Long-Term Prognostic Risk After Neoadjuvant Chemotherapy Associated With Residual Cancer Burden and Breast Cancer Subtype. *Journal of clinical oncology : official journal of the American Society of Clinical Oncology* **35**, 1049-1060 (2017).

223.   Steward, L., Conant, L., Gao, F. & Margenthaler, J.A. Predictive Factors and Patterns of Recurrence in Patients with Triple Negative Breast Cancer. *Annals of Surgical Oncology* **21**, 2165-2171 (2014).

224.   Kather, J.N., *et al.* Topography of cancer-associated immune cells in human solid tumors. *Elife* **7**(2018).

225.   Pollard, J.W. Tumour-educated macrophages promote tumour progression and metastasis. *Nature Reviews Cancer* **4**, 71-78 (2004).

226.   Wyckoff, J., *et al.* A Paracrine Loop between Tumor Cells and Macrophages Is Required for Tumor Cell Migration in Mammary Tumors. *Cancer Res* **64**, 7022 (2004).

227.   Gao, M.-Q., *et al.* Stromal fibroblasts from the interface zone of human breast carcinomas induce an epithelial–mesenchymal transition-like state in breast cancer cells in vitro. *Journal of Cell Science* **123**, 3507 (2010).

228.   Van Berckelaer, C., *et al.* The spatial localization of CD163+ tumor-associated macrophages predicts prognosis and response to therapy in inflammatory breast cancer. *Journal of Clinical Oncology* **38**, 3086-3086 (2020).

229.   Ch'ng, E.S., Tuan Sharif, S.E. & Jaafar, H. In human invasive breast ductal carcinoma, tumor stromal macrophages and tumor nest macrophages have distinct relationships with clinicopathological parameters and tumor angiogenesis. *Virchows Archiv* **462**, 257-267 (2013).

230.   Gruosso, T., *et al.* Spatially distinct tumor immune microenvironments stratify triple-negative breast cancers. *J Clin Invest* **129**, 1785-1800 (2019).

231.   König, L., *et al.* Dissimilar patterns of tumor-infiltrating immune cells at the invasive tumor front and tumor center are associated with response to neoadjuvant chemotherapy in primary breast cancer. *BMC Cancer* **19**, 120 (2019).

232.   Schrörs, B., *et al.* Multi-Omics Characterization of the 4T1 Murine Mammary Gland Tumor Model. *Frontiers in Oncology* **10**(2020).

233.   Tao, K., Fang, M., Alroy, J. & Sahagian, G.G. Imagable 4T1 model for the study of late stage breast cancer. *BMC Cancer* **8**, 228 (2008).

234.   Urtreger, A., *et al.* Modulation of fibronectin expression and proteolytic activity associated with the invasive and metastatic phenotype in two new murine mammary tumor cell lines. *International Journal of Oncology* **11**, 489-496 (1997).

235.   Liu, Y. & Cao, X. Characteristics and Significance of the Pre-metastatic Niche. *Cancer Cell* **30**, 668-681 (2016).

236.   Le Mercier, I., *et al.* Tumor promotion by intratumoral plasmacytoid dendritic cells is reversed by TLR7 ligand treatment. *Cancer Res* **73**, 4629-4640 (2013).

237.   Veglia, F. & Gabrilovich, D.I. Dendritic cells in cancer: the role revisited. *Current opinion in immunology* **45**, 43-51 (2017).

238.   Cobaleda, C., Schebesta, A., Delogu, A. & Busslinger, M. Pax5: the guardian of B cell identity and function. *Nature Immunology* **8**, 463-470 (2007).

239.   Cheung, Kevin J., Gabrielson, E., Werb, Z. & Ewald, Andrew J. Collective Invasion in Breast Cancer Requires a Conserved Basal Epithelial Program. *Cell* **155**, 1639-1651 (2013).

240.   Porter, R.J., Murray, G.I. & McLean, M.H. Current concepts in tumour-derived organoids. *Br J Cancer* **123**, 1209-1218 (2020).

241.   Padmanaban, V., *et al.* E-cadherin is required for metastasis in multiple models of breast cancer. *Nature* **573**, 439-444 (2019).

242.   Nguyen-Ngoc, K.-V., *et al.* ECM microenvironment regulates collective migration and local dissemination in normal and malignant mammary epithelium. *Proceedings of the National Academy of Sciences* **109**, E2595 (2012).

243.   Zhou, X., *et al.* Activation of the Akt/Mammalian Target of Rapamycin/4E-BP1 Pathway by ErbB2 Overexpression Predicts Tumor Progression in Breast Cancers. *Clinical Cancer Research* **10**, 6779 (2004).

244.   Lee, H. Phosphorylated mTOR Expression Profiles in Human Normal and Carcinoma Tissues. *Disease Markers* **2017**, 1397063 (2017).

245.   Düvel, K., *et al.* Activation of a Metabolic Gene Regulatory Network Downstream of mTOR Complex 1. *Molecular Cell* **39**, 171-183 (2010).

246.   Hoffmann, C., *et al.* Hypoxia promotes breast cancer cell invasion through HIF-1α-mediated up-regulation of the invadopodial actin bundling protein CSRP2. *Scientific reports* **8**, 10191-10191 (2018).

247.   Chaturvedi, P., *et al.* Hypoxia-inducible factor-dependent breast cancer-mesenchymal stem cell bidirectional signaling promotes metastasis. *J Clin Invest* **123**, 189-205 (2013).

248.   Liu, Z.-J., Semenza, G.L. & Zhang, H.-F. Hypoxia-inducible factor 1 and breast cancer metastasis. *J Zhejiang Univ Sci B* **16**, 32-43 (2015).

249.   Morris, A. & Möller, G. Regulation of Cellular Antibody Synthesis. *The Journal of Immunology* **101**, 439 (1968).

250.   Mauri, C. & Ehrenstein, M.R. The 'short' history of regulatory B cells. *Trends in Immunology* **29**, 34-40 (2008).

251.   Vézina, C., Kudelski, A. & Sehgal, S.N. Rapamycin (AY-22,989), a new antifungal antibiotic. I. Taxonomy of the producing streptomycete and isolation of the active principle. *J Antibiot (Tokyo)* **28**, 721-726 (1975).

252.   Brown, E.J., *et al.* A mammalian protein targeted by G1-arresting rapamycin–receptor complex. *Nature* **369**, 756-758 (1994).

253. Sabatini, D.M., Erdjument-Bromage, H., Lui, M., Tempst, P. & Snyder, S.H. RAFT1: A mammalian protein that binds to FKBP12 in a rapamycin-dependent fashion and is homologous to yeast TORs. *Cell* **78**, 35-43 (1994).

254. Liu, G.Y. & Sabatini, D.M. mTOR at the nexus of nutrition, growth, ageing and disease. *Nature Reviews Molecular Cell Biology* **21**, 183-203 (2020).

255. Zhou, H. & Huang, S. Role of mTOR signaling in tumor cell motility, invasion and metastasis. *Curr Protein Pept Sci* **12**, 30-42 (2011).

256. Figueiredo, V.C., Markworth, J.F. & Cameron-Smith, D. Considerations on mTOR regulation at serine 2448: implications for muscle metabolism studies. *Cellular and Molecular Life Sciences* **74**, 2537-2545 (2017).

257. Chiang, G.G. & Abraham, R.T. Phosphorylation of Mammalian Target of Rapamycin (mTOR) at Ser-2448 IsMediated by p70S6 Kinase*. *Journal of Biological Chemistry* **280**, 25485-25490 (2005).

258. Bose, S., Chandran, S., Mirocha, J.M. & Bose, N. The Akt pathway in human breast cancer: a tissue-array-based analysis. *Mod Pathol* **19**, 238-245 (2006).

259. Ma, B.L., *et al.* Immunohistochemical analysis of phosphorylated mammalian target of rapamycin and its downstream signaling components in invasive breast cancer. *Mol Med Rep* **12**, 5246-5254 (2015).

260. Ueng, S.-H., *et al.* Phosphorylated mTOR expression correlates with poor outcome in early-stage triple negative breast carcinomas. *Int J Clin Exp Pathol* **5**, 806-813 (2012).

261. Walsh, S., *et al.* mTOR in breast cancer: Differential expression in triple-negative and non-triple-negative tumors. *The Breast* **21**, 178-182 (2012).

262. Montero, J.C., *et al.* Active kinase profiling, genetic and pharmacological data define mTOR as an important common target in triple-negative breast cancer. *Oncogene* **33**, 148-156 (2014).

263. Liu, L., *et al.* Rapamycin inhibits cell motility by suppression of mTOR-mediated S6K1 and 4E-BP1 pathways. *Oncogene* **25**, 7029-7040 (2006).

264. Chen, M.-B., *et al.* MicroRNA-451 regulates AMPK/mTORC1 signaling and fascin1 expression in HT-29 colorectal cancer. *Cellular Signalling* **26**, 102-109 (2014).

265. Liu, H., *et al.* Fascin actin-bundling protein 1 in human cancer: Promising biomarker or therapeutic target? *Molecular Therapy - Oncolytics* **20**, 240-264 (2021).

266. Lamouille, S. & Derynck, R. Cell size and invasion in TGF-beta-induced epithelial to mesenchymal transition is regulated by activation of the mTOR pathway. *J Cell Biol* **178**, 437-451 (2007).

267.	Liu, L., Chen, L., Chung, J. & Huang, S. Rapamycin inhibits F-actin reorganization and phosphorylation of focal adhesion proteins. *Oncogene* **27**, 4998-5010 (2008).

268.	Liu, L., *et al.* Proliferation, migration and invasion of triple negative breast cancer cells are suppressed by berbamine via the PI3K/Akt/MDM2/p53 and PI3K/Akt/mTOR signaling pathways. *Oncol Lett* **21**, 70-70 (2021).

269.	Chen, Y., Wei, H., Liu, F. & Guan, J.L. Hyperactivation of mammalian target of rapamycin complex 1 (mTORC1) promotes breast cancer progression through enhancing glucose starvation-induced autophagy and Akt signaling. *J Biol Chem* **289**, 1164-1173 (2014).

270.	Jacinto, E., *et al.* Mammalian TOR complex 2 controls the actin cytoskeleton and is rapamycin insensitive. *Nat Cell Biol* **6**, 1122-1128 (2004).

271.	Serrano, I., McDonald, P.C., Lock, F.E. & Dedhar, S. Role of the integrin-linked kinase (ILK)/Rictor complex in TGFβ-1-induced epithelial–mesenchymal transition (EMT). *Oncogene* **32**, 50-60 (2013).

272.	Ross, S.H. & Cantrell, D.A. Signaling and Function of Interleukin-2 in T Lymphocytes. *Annual review of immunology* **36**, 411-433 (2018).

273.	Junttila, I.S. Tuning the Cytokine Responses: An Update on Interleukin (IL)-4 and IL-13 Receptor Complexes. *Front Immunol* **9**(2018).

274.	Pinno, J., *et al.* Interleukin-6 influences stress-signalling by reducing the expression of the mTOR-inhibitor REDD1 in a STAT3-dependent manner. *Cell Signal* **28**, 907-916 (2016).

275.	Wang, H., *et al.* IL-12 Influence mTOR to Modulate CD8(+) T Cells Differentiation through T-bet and Eomesodermin in Response to Invasive Pulmonary Aspergillosis. *Int J Med Sci* **14**, 977-983 (2017).

276.	Lamouille, S., Connolly, E., Smyth, J.W., Akhurst, R.J. & Derynck, R. TGF-β-induced activation of mTOR complex 2 drives epithelial-mesenchymal transition and cell invasion. *Journal of cell science* **125**, 1259-1273 (2012).

277.	Zhou, J.X., Fan, L.X., Li, X., Calvet, J.P. & Li, X. TNFα signaling regulates cystic epithelial cell proliferation through Akt/mTOR and ERK/MAPK/Cdk2 mediated Id2 signaling. *PLoS One* **10**, e0131043 (2015).

278.	Deason, K., *et al.* BCAP links IL-1R to the PI3K-mTOR pathway and regulates pathogenic Th17 cell differentiation. *J Exp Med* **215**, 2413-2428 (2018).

279.	Jia, Q.-N. & Zeng, Y.-P. Rapamycin blocks the IL-13-induced deficiency of Epidermal Barrier Related Proteins via upregulation of miR-143 in HaCaT Keratinocytes. in *International journal of medical sciences*, Vol. 17 2087-2094 (2020).

280. Sharma, G., *et al.* IL-27 inhibits IFN-γ induced autophagy by concomitant induction of JAK/PI3 K/Akt/mTOR cascade and up-regulation of Mcl-1 in Mycobacterium tuberculosis H37Rv infected macrophages. *The International Journal of Biochemistry & Cell Biology* **55**, 335-347 (2014).

281. Floyd, S., *et al.* The insulin-like growth factor-I-mTOR signaling pathway induces the mitochondrial pyrimidine nucleotide carrier to promote cell growth. *Mol Biol Cell* **18**, 3545-3555 (2007).

282. Trinh, X.B., *et al.* The VEGF pathway and the AKT/mTOR/p70S6K1 signalling pathway in human epithelial ovarian cancer. *Br J Cancer* **100**, 971-978 (2009).

283. Razmara, M., Heldin, C.H. & Lennartsson, J. Platelet-derived growth factor-induced Akt phosphorylation requires mTOR/Rictor and phospholipase C-γ1, whereas S6 phosphorylation depends on mTOR/Raptor and phospholipase D. *Cell Commun Signal* **11**, 3 (2013).

284. Lee, H., Na, K.J. & Choi, H. Differences in Tumor Immune Microenvironment in Metastatic Sites of Breast Cancer. *Frontiers in Oncology* **11**(2021).

285. Zhu, L., *et al.* Metastatic breast cancers have reduced immune cell recruitment but harbor increased macrophages relative to their matched primary tumors. *Journal for ImmunoTherapy of Cancer* **7**, 265 (2019).

286. Morrison Joly, M., *et al.* Two distinct mTORC2-dependent pathways converge on Rac1 to drive breast cancer metastasis. *Breast Cancer Research* **19**, 74 (2017).

287. Zhang, H., *et al.* Patient-derived xenografts of triple-negative breast cancer reproduce molecular features of patient tumors and respond to mTOR inhibition. *Breast Cancer Research* **16**, R36 (2014).

288. Zhang, W., *et al.* Aurora-A/ERK1/2/mTOR axis promotes tumor progression in triple-negative breast cancer and dual-targeting Aurora-A/mTOR shows synthetic lethality. *Cell death & disease* **10**, 606 (2019).

289. Mateo, F., *et al.* Stem cell-like transcriptional reprogramming mediates metastatic resistance to mTOR inhibition. *Oncogene* **36**, 2737-2749 (2017).

290. Kwon, Y.S., *et al.* Metformin selectively targets 4T1 tumorspheres and enhances the antitumor effects of doxorubicin by downregulating the AKT and STAT3 signaling pathways. *Oncol Lett* **17**, 2523-2530 (2019).

291. Rinaldi, G., *et al.* In Vivo Evidence for Serine Biosynthesis-Defined Sensitivity of Lung Metastasis, but Not of Primary Breast Tumors, to mTORC1 Inhibition. *Molecular Cell* **81**, 386-397.e387 (2021).

292. Lin, T.-J., *et al.* Rapamycin Promotes Mouse 4T1 Tumor Metastasis that Can Be Reversed by a Dendritic Cell-Based Vaccine. *PLoS One* **10**, e0138335-e0138335 (2015).

293. Langdon, S., *et al.* Combination of dual mTORC1/2 inhibition and immune-checkpoint blockade potentiates anti-tumour immunity. *Oncoimmunology* **7**, e1458810-e1458810 (2018).

294. Rodrik-Outmezguine, V.S., *et al.* Overcoming mTOR resistance mutations with a new-generation mTOR inhibitor. *Nature* **534**, 272-276 (2016).

295. Kuroshima, K., *et al.* Potential new therapy of Rapalink-1, a new generation mammalian target of rapamycin inhibitor, against sunitinib-resistant renal cell carcinoma. *Cancer Sci* **111**, 1607-1618 (2020).

296. Hasskarl, J. Everolimus. in *Small Molecules in Oncology* (ed. Martens, U.M.) 101-123 (Springer International Publishing, Cham, 2018).

297. Baselga, J., *et al.* Everolimus in postmenopausal hormone-receptor-positive advanced breast cancer. *The New England journal of medicine* **366**, 520-529 (2012).

298. Singh, J.C., *et al.* Phase 2 trial of everolimus and carboplatin combination in patients with triple negative metastatic breast cancer. *Breast Cancer Research* **16**, R32 (2014).

299. Temsirolimus Plus Neratinib for Patients With Metastatic HER2-Amplified or Triple Negative Breast Cancer. (https://ClinicalTrials.gov/show/NCT01111825).

300. mTORC1/2 Inhibitor AZD2014 or the Oral AKT Inhibitor AZD5363 for Recurrent Endometrial and Ovarian. (https://ClinicalTrials.gov/show/NCT02208375).

301. A Study of AZD2014 in Combination With Selumetinib in Patients With Advanced Cancers. (https://ClinicalTrials.gov/show/NCT02583542).

302. PQR309 and Eribulin in Metastatic HER2 Negative and Triple-negative Breast Cancer (PIQHASSO). (https://ClinicalTrials.gov/show/NCT02723877).

303. Lee, J.S., *et al.* Phase I clinical trial of the combination of eribulin and everolimus in patients with metastatic triple-negative breast cancer. *Breast Cancer Research* **21**, 119 (2019).

304. Hu, Q., *et al.* Atlas of breast cancer infiltrated B-lymphocytes revealed by paired single-cell RNA-sequencing and antigen receptor profiling. *Nat Commun* **12**, 2186 (2021).

305. Ong, C.-A.J., *et al.* An Optimised Protocol Harnessing Laser Capture Microdissection for Transcriptomic Analysis on Matched Primary and Metastatic Colorectal Tumours. *Scientific Reports* **10**, 682 (2020).

306. Burkholder, T., Foltz, C., Karlsson, E., Linton, C.G. & Smith, J.M. Health Evaluation of Experimental Laboratory Mice. *Curr Protoc Mouse Biol* **2**, 145-165 (2012).

307. Livak, K.J. & Schmittgen, T.D. Analysis of relative gene expression data using real-time quantitative PCR and the 2(-Delta Delta C(T)) Method. *Methods* **25**, 402-408 (2001).

308.   Dexter, D.L., *et al.* Heterogeneity of Tumor Cells from a Single Mouse Mammary Tumor. *Cancer Res* **38**, 3174 (1978).

309.   Hendry, S., *et al.* Assessing Tumor-infiltrating Lymphocytes in Solid Tumors: A Practical Review for Pathologists and Proposal for a Standardized Method From the International Immunooncology Biomarkers Working Group: Part 1: Assessing the Host Immune Response, TILs in Invasive Breast Carcinoma and Ductal Carcinoma In Situ, Metastatic Tumor Deposits and Areas for Further Research. *Advances in anatomic pathology* **24**, 235-251 (2017).

310.   Nguyen-Ngoc, K.V., *et al.* 3D culture assays of murine mammary branching morphogenesis and epithelial invasion. *Methods Mol Biol* **1189**, 135-162 (2015).

311.   Cattaneo, C.M., *et al.* Tumor organoid-T-cell coculture systems. *Nat Protoc* **15**, 15-39 (2020).

312.   Amigó, M., Payá, M., De Rosa, S. & Terencio, M.C. Antipsoriatic effects of avarol-3'-thiosalicylate are mediated by inhibition of TNF-alpha generation and NF-kappaB activation in mouse skin. *Br J Pharmacol* **152**, 353-365 (2007).